D1234262

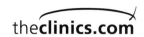

FOOT AND
ANKLE CLINICS

Rheumatoid Arthritis in Foot and Ankle Surgery

GUEST EDITOR
Clifford L. Jeng, MD

CONSULTING EDITOR
Mark S. Myerson, MD

September 2007 • Volume 12 • Number 3

SAUNDERS

An Imprint of Elsevier, Inc.
PHILADELPHIA   LONDON   TORONTO   MONTREAL   SYDNEY   TOKYO

W.B. SAUNDERS COMPANY
A Division of Elsevier Inc.

1600 John F. Kennedy Blvd., Suite 1800, Philadelphia, PA 19103-2899

http://www.theclinics.com

FOOT AND ANKLE CLINICS

September 2007

Editor: Debora Dellapena

Volume 12, Number 3
ISSN 1083-7515
ISBN 1-4160-5070-1
978-1-4160-5070-4

Copyright © 2007 by Elsevier Inc. All rights reserved. No part of this publication may be reproduced or transmitted in any form or by any means, electronic or mechanical, including photocopy, recording, or any information retrieval system, without written permission from the Publisher.

Single photocopies of single articles may be made for personal use as allowed by national copyright laws. Permission of the publisher and payment of a fee is required for all other photocopying, including multiple or systematic copying, copying for advertising or promotional purposes, resale, and all forms of document delivery. Special rates are available for educational institutions that wish to make photocopies for nonprofit educational classroom use. Permission may be sought directly from Elsevier's Global Rights Department in Oxford, UK: phone: 215-239-3804 or +44 (0) 1865 843830, fax: +44 (0) 1865 853333, e-mail: healthpermissions@elsevier.com. Requests may also be completed online via the Elsevier homepage (http://www.elsevier.com/permissions). In the USA, users may clear permissions and make payments through the Copyright Clearance Center, Inc., 222 Rosewood Drive, Danvers, MA 01923, USA; phone: (978) 750-8400, fax: (978) 750-4744, and in the UK through the Copyright Licensing Agency Rapid Clearance Service (CLARCS), 90 Tottenham Court Road, London WIP 0LP, UK; phone (+44) 171 436 5931; fax: (+44) 171 436 3986. Other countries may have a local reprographic rights agency for payments.

Reprints. For copies of 100 or more of articles in this publication, please contact the Commercial Reprints Department, Elsevier Inc., 360 Park Avenue South, New York, New York 10010-1710. Tel.: (212) 633-3813; Fax: (212) 462-1935, e-mail: reprints@elsevier.com

The ideas and opinions expressed in *Foot and Ankle Clinics* do not necessarily reflect those of the Publisher. The Publisher does not assume any responsibility for any injury and/or damage to persons or property arising out of or related to any use of the material contained in this periodical. The reader is advised to check the appropriate medical literature and the product information currently provided by the manufacturer of each drug to be administered to verify the dosage, the method and duration of administration, or contraindications. It is the responsibility of the treating physician or other health care professional, relying on independent experience and knowledge of the patient, to determine drug dosages and the best treatment for the patient. Mention of any product in this issue should not be construed as endorsement by the contributors, editors, or the Publisher of the product or manufacturers' claims.

Foot and Ankle Clinics (ISSN 1083-7515) is published quarterly by Elsevier, Inc., 360 Park Avenue South, New York, NY 10010-1710. Months of issue are March, June, September, and December. Business and Editorial Offices: 1600 John F. Kennedy Blvd., Suite 1800, Philadelphia, PA 19103-2899. Customer Service Office: 6277 Sea Harbor Drive, Orlando, FL 32887-4800. Periodicals postage paid at New York, NY, and additional mailing offices. Subscription prices are $314.00 per year Institutional, $270.00 per year Institutional USA, $314.00 per year Institutional Canada, $253.00 per year Personal, $187.00 per year Personal USA, $209.00 per year Personal Canada, $121.00 per year Personal student, $94.00 per year Personal student USA, $121.00 per year Personal student Canada. To receive student/resident rate, orders must be accompanied by name of affiliated institution, date of term, and the *signature* of program/residency coordinator on institution letterhead. Orders will be billed at individual rate until proof of status is received. Foreign air speed delivery is included in all *Clinics* subscription prices. All prices are subject to change without notice. POSTMASTER: Send address changes to *Foot and Ankle Clinics*, Elsevier Periodicals Customer Service, 6277 Sea Harbor Drive, Orlando, FL 32887-4800. **Customer Service: 1-800-654-2452 (US). From outside of the US, call 1-407-345-1000.**

Printed in the United States of America.

CONSULTING EDITOR

MARK S. MYERSON, MD, Medical Director, The Institute for Foot and Ankle Reconstructive Surgery, Mercy Medical Center, Baltimore, Maryland

GUEST EDITOR

CLIFFORD L. JENG, MD, Foot and Ankle Institute, Mercy Medical Center, Baltimore, Maryland

CONTRIBUTORS

JOHN G. ANDERSON, MD, Associate Professor, Department of Orthopaedic Surgery, College of Human Medicine, Michigan State University, Grand Rapids; and Orthopaedic Associates of Grand Rapids, P.C., Foot and Ankle Division, Grand Rapids, Michigan

MICHAEL S. ARONOW, MD, Associate Professor, Department of Orthopaedic Surgery, University of Connecticut Health Center, Farmington, Connecticut

LOUIS SAMUEL BAROUK, MD, Polyclinique de Bourdeaux, Bordeaux, France

PIERRE BAROUK, MD, Clinique St. Antoine de Padoue, Bordeaux, France

CHRISTOPHER BIBBO, DO, DPM, FACS, FAAOS, FACFAS, Chief, Foot and Ankle Section; Director, Foot and Ankle Service, Department of Orthopedics, Marshfield Clinic, Marshfield; Clinical Instructor, Department of Orthopedics and Rehabilitation, University of Wisconsin Medical School, Madison, Wisconsin

DONALD R. BOHAY, MD, Associate Professor, Department of Orthopaedic Surgery, College of Human Medicine, Michigan State University, Grand Rapids; and Orthopaedic Associates of Grand Rapids, P.C., Foot and Ankle Division, Grand Rapids, Michigan

LOUISE A. CRAWFORD, MB, ChB, MRSC (Ed), Specialist Registrar, Wrightington Hospital, Wigan, United Kingdom

MARIAM HAKIM-ZARGAR, MPH, MD, Fellow, Department of Orthopaedic Surgery, John Dempsey Hospital, Farmington, Connecticut

G. HOLT, MRCS, Specialist Registrar, Trauma and Orthopaedic Surgery, West of Scotland Deanery, Department of Orthopaedic and Trauma Surgery, Glasgow Royal Infirmary, Glasgow, United Kingdom

ANN KENYON, BSc, MA, Researcher, Wrightington Hospital, Wigan, United Kingdom

C. SENTHIL KUMAR, FRCS(Tr&Orth), Consultant Orthopaedic Surgeon, Department of Orthopaedic and Trauma Surgery, Glasgow Royal Infirmary, Glasgow, United Kingdom

MARLYN LORENZO, MD, FACR, Mercy Medical Center, Baltimore, Maryland

ANDREW P. MOLLOY, MBChB, FRCS(Tr&Orth), Fellow, The Institute for Foot and Ankle Reconstructive Surgery, Mercy Medical Center, Baltimore, Maryland

MARK S. MYERSON, MD, Medical Director, The Institute for Foot and Ankle Reconstructive Surgery, Mercy Medical Center, Baltimore, Maryland

VINCENT JAMES SAMMARCO, MD, Cincinnati Sports Medicine and Orthopaedic Center, Cincinnati, Ohio

BENJAMIN W. STEVENS, MD, Resident Physician, Grand Rapids Medical Education and Research Center, Michigan State University, Orthopaedic Surgery Residency Program, Grand Rapids, Michigan

RAJEEV SUNEJA, MS(Orth), MSc(Tr), FRCS(Tr&Orth), Foot and Ankle Fellow, Wrightington Hospital, Wigan, United Kingdom

PETER L.R. WOOD, MB, BS, FRCS, Consultant Orthopaedic Surgeon, Wrightington Hospital, Wigan, United Kingdom

CONTENTS

> Forefoot problems in patients who have rheumatoid arthritis are
> common. The progressive joint destruction causes a redistribution
> of weight about the forefoot, with a diminished weightbearing
> capacity of the first metatarsophalangeal (MTP) joint. Changes
> around the first MTP joint include synovitis, joint instability with
> subluxation, and arthritic change. Hallux MTP fusion in patients
> who have rheumatoid arthritis acts to permanently restore align-
> ment and restore the medial column support of the foot, while at
> the same time enabling the first MTP to resume its original
> weightbearing role. Rheumatoid hallux MTP fusion and its
> rationale are reviewed.

> Surgical options for treatment of the hallux valgus deformity in the
> rheumatoid forefoot are numerous, but long-term results of many
> of these procedures have been less than satisfactory. Controversy

exists as to whether excision or fusion is preferred for the treatment of the hallux metatarsophalangeal (MTP) joint. The role of replacement arthroplasty needs to be evaluated. The available surgical options for treatment of the arthritic first MTP joint in rheumatoid arthritis include arthrodesis, excision of the metatarsal head with or without interposition of the soft tissues, excision of the proximal phalanx, and silicone hinge replacement. This article discusses the various types of arthroplasty of the first MTP joint and the reported outcomes in the rheumatoid forefoot.

This review article discusses the pathologic and anatomic basis of rheumatoid lesser toe deformities. It covers the history of lesser metatarsal head resection being used in its treatment and the theoretic basis behind differing techniques and their relative results and complications. The authors also present their preferred technique for lesser metatarsal head resection.

The authors propose a joint-preserving surgery for rheumatoid forefoot deformities as an alternative to the "classic" surgical approach to the rheumatoid forefoot. The main principle is joint preservation by shortening osteotomies of all the metatarsals performed at the primary location of the rheumatoid forefoot lesions, namely the metatarsophalangeal (MTP) joints and metatarsal heads. A scarf osteotomy is normally performed on the first ray. A Weil osteotomy is performed on the lesser metatarsals. Excellent correction of the hallux valgus deformity in the rheumatoid forefoot can be achieved with a scarf osteotomy in 92% of cases without the need for MTP joint arthrodesis. Similarly, 86% of the lateral metatarsal heads can be preserved using Weil osteotomies.

There is a wide variety of hindfoot disease seen in patients with rheumatoid arthritis. Initial treatment is conservative including optimizing medical management to control the disease process. Should symptoms persist, surgical treatment may be performed, although there is an increased complication rate related to both the disease and the side effects of the medications used to treat it.

FORTHCOMING ISSUES

RECENT ISSUES

THE CLINICS ARE NOW AVAILABLE ONLINE!

http://www.theclinics.com

ELSEVIER SAUNDERS

Foot Ankle Clin N Am
12 (2007) ix–x

FOOT AND ANKLE CLINICS

Foreword

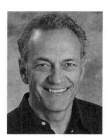

Mark S. Myerson, MD
Consulting Editor

It is quite interesting how some surgeries of the foot and ankle have stood the test of time, whereas others have either been abandoned or improved upon. Management of arthritis and deformity of the foot and ankle in the patient with rheumatoid arthritis has indeed evolved in many respects; yet some procedures, such as reconstruction of the forefoot, have not changed very much.

Although there remain proponents of implant or resection arthroplasty of the hallux metatarsophalangeal (MP) joint, the results of arthrodesis have been consistent over the decades, and this remains the ideal procedure for correction of arthritis and deformity. Clearly, the disadvantage of arthrodesis is the increased load on the interphalangeal joint, and unless the fusion is positioned correctly, the latter will occur with an increased frequency. The hallux should be slightly more supinated and placed in slightly more of a neutral position than normal, but left in the appropriate amount of dorsiflexion to avoid loading of the interphalangeal joint. It is certainly feasible to perform joint-sparing surgery on the hallux, and where erosive changes are present in the lesser toe MP joints with a normally aligned hallux, then either a shortening osteotomy, bunionectomy, or nothing is done to the hallux. If the hallux is left alone while the lesser metatarsals are shortened or the heads removed, there is an increased load on the hallux, which indeed may drift into valgus in time. However, the joint should be spared from arthrodesis if entirely normal in appearance.

The article by Barouk is quite fascinating. The results he has obtained with joint preservation in the rheumatoid forefoot are quite astounding,

1083-7515/07/$ - see front matter © 2007 Elsevier Inc. All rights reserved.
doi:10.1016/j.fcl.2007.06.001

but unfortunately many surgeons have not been able to duplicate these results predictably, and metatarsal head resection with arthrodesis of the hallux MP joint has remained the more reliable procedure. With all rheumatoid forefoot surgery, perfusion of the skin and toes postoperatively is important, and intraoperative manipulation with excessive retraction and pinching of the skin should be avoided. In addition to fragility of the skin, vasculitis may be present, and this combined with peripheral vascular disease places the patient at increased risk for ischemic complications. For this reason, I prefer to operate on the rheumatoid forefoot without a tourniquet, or at the least check the perfusion to the toes periodically during the surgery; if k-wires are used, I use the smallest diameter k-wire possible to avoid ischemia of the toes. The options for hindfoot and ankle correction have not changed very much.

Although there are advocates of isolated hindfoot joint arthrodesis, it is worth remembering that a triple arthrodesis in these patients is extremely reliable, which in my hands is the preferred procedure. However, if the deformity is severe, and the hindfoot is fixed in marked valgus, a medial approach to perform the arthrodesis may be preferable to avoid the potential for wound dehiscence when straightening the hindfoot valgus.

Mark S. Myerson, MD
Institute for Foot and Ankle Reconstruction at Mercy Medical Center
301 St. Paul Place
Baltimore, MD 21202, USA

E-mail address: mark4feet@aol.com

**ELSEVIER
SAUNDERS**

Foot Ankle Clin N Am
12 (2007) xi

**FOOT AND
ANKLE CLINICS**

Dedication

I would like to dedicate this issue to my parents who first gave me life, to my wife who constantly nurtures it, to my two children who give it purpose, and to Roger Mann who taught me to use these two clumsy appendages.

Clifford L. Jeng, MD
*Foot and Ankle Institute
Mercy Medical Center
301 Saint Paul Place
Baltimore, MD 21202*

E-mail address: cjeng@mdmercy.com

1083-7515/07/$ - see front matter © 2007 Elsevier Inc. All rights reserved.
doi:10.1016/j.fcl.2007.05.005

ELSEVIER
SAUNDERS

Foot Ankle Clin N Am
12 (2007) xiii–xiv

FOOT AND
ANKLE CLINICS

Preface

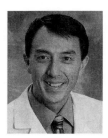

Clifford L. Jeng, MD
Guest Editor

Rheumatoid arthritis affects approximately 1% of the population, with a greater prevalence in women than in men. Orthopedic surgeons are frequently consulted regarding management of painful arthritis and deformity in these patients. In the hip and knee joint, prosthetic arthroplasty has enjoyed success rates similar to those in patients who have noninflammatory arthritis. In the foot and ankle, however, surgical treatment traditionally has centered on arthrodesis of the involved joints.

During the past decade the management of rheumatoid foot and ankle problems has evolved significantly, with newer joint-sparing techniques in both the ankle and forefoot that may potentially improve function and quality of life. There have also been major advances in the medical treatment of rheumatoid arthritis, particularly with the introduction of anti–tumor necrosis factor drug therapy.

The purpose of this issue of *Foot and Ankle Clinics* is to update surgeons on the current thinking in the management of rheumatoid foot and ankle problems from experts in their respective fields worldwide. We have invited our esteemed colleagues from England and France to review the results of total ankle replacement in rheumatoid arthritis, and the techniques of resection arthroplasty, prosthetic arthroplasty, and shortening osteotomy in the reconstruction of rheumatoid forefoot deformities. American surgeons have been enlisted to cover the latest trends in arthrodesis surgery of the ankle, hindfoot, and forefoot. We have included an article that addresses the perioperative risks of wound-healing problems and infection associated with the various disease-modifying antirheumatic drugs. The final article is an

1083-7515/07/$ - see front matter © 2007 Elsevier Inc. All rights reserved.
doi:10.1016/j.fcl.2007.05.004

foot.theclinics.com

up-to-date rheumatology primer that includes a concise discussion of the newer tumor necrosis factor inhibitor drugs and an update on the relative risks of the COX-2 nonsteroidal anti-inflammatory drugs versus the nonselective nonsteroidal anti-inflammatory drugs.

Our hope is that this issue will provide an improved knowledge base that will enable us collectively as orthopedic surgeons, collectively to provide better care for our patients who are afflicted with this disabling disease.

Clifford L. Jeng, MD
Foot and Ankle Institute
Mercy Medical Center
301 Saint Paul Place
Baltimore, MD 21202

E-mail address: cjeng@mdmercy.com

ELSEVIER
SAUNDERS

Foot Ankle Clin N Am
12 (2007) 395–404

FOOT AND
ANKLE CLINICS

Hallux Metatarsophalangeal Joint Fusion for the Rheumatoid Forefoot

Benjamin W. Stevens, MD[a,*],
John G. Anderson, MD[b,c],
Donald R. Bohay, MD[b,c]

[a]Grand Rapids Medical Education and Research Center/Michigan State University
Orthopaedic Surgery Residency Program, 300 Lafayette,
Suite 3400, Grand Rapids, MI 49503, USA
[b]Department of Orthopaedic Surgery, College of Human Medicine,
Michigan State University, East Lansing, MI 48824-1316, USA
[c]Orthopaedic Associates of Grand Rapids P. C., Foot and Ankle Division,
1111 Leffingwell NE, Suite 100, Grand Rapids, MI 49525, USA

Rheumatoid arthritis can begin in the foot in nearly 20% of cases and generally affects the forefoot more commonly than the hindfoot [1]. Chronic synovitis leads to a severe deformity of the foot that can be clinically apparent in nearly all patients who have a 10-year history of the disease [2]. This deformity invariably leads to disruption of the foot's intrinsic tripod stability and ultimately a disabling gait.

In the past, after failed conservative treatment of rheumatoid hallux pathology, operative interventions have varied greatly. This article addresses arthrodesis of the hallux metatarsophalangeal (MTP) joint and its role in restoring the weightbearing function of the medial column and first MTP joint.

Anatomy

The MTP joint of the hallux is much more complex than the lateral MTP joints, because one third of the body weight is supported through the two sesamoids [3]. The first MTP joint functions primarily in the sagittal plane, providing for dorsiflexion and plantarflexion. Sliding, rolling, and

---

* Corresponding author.
E-mail address: bw_stevens@hotmail.com (B.W. Stevens).

1083-7515/07/$ - see front matter © 2007 Elsevier Inc. All rights reserved.
doi:10.1016/j.fcl.2007.04.003

compression take place, but abduction and adduction are limited. Multiple centers of motion about the first MTP joint have been described [4]. The capsuloligamentous–sesamoid complex provides most of the stability to the joint, because the proximal phalanx exhibits only a shallow articular surface. Collateral ligaments, metatarsosesamoid suspensory ligaments, an intersesamoid ligament, and the plantar plate provide marked support also. This capsuloligamentous structure is combined with the tendons of the flexor and extensor hallucis brevis, adductor brevis, and the adductor hallucis tendons (Fig. 1) [1].

Biomechanics

The functional requirements of the hallux MTP joint imply the need for great stability. As part of the critical tripod of the foot, it supports twice the load of the lesser toes. Forces acting across this joint can reach 40% to 60% of body weight, with nearly eight times body weight experienced during a running jump [4].

The hallux rests in a mean position of 16° of dorsiflexion, with a passive arc of motion ranging from 3° to 43° of plantarflexion and from 40° to 100° of dorsiflexion. Incorporated in dorsiflexion is the windlass mechanism. As first described by Hicks [5], the plantar aponeurosis tension is increased with dorsiflexion of the toes. As the toes dorsiflex, the proximal phalangeal insertion of the aponeurosis winds the fascia around the metatarsal heads, thus creating tension and raising the medial arch (Fig. 2). This in turn provides passive stabilization of the medial column, especially during push-off. Ten degrees of plantarflexion of the first ray is noted [5]. Recently Lombardi and colleagues [6] examined the effect of first MTP fusion on the sagittal position of the medial arch and first ray. They concluded that hallux

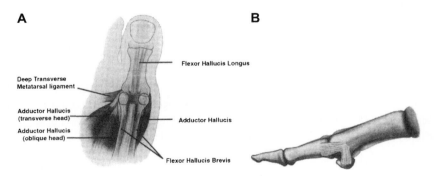

Fig. 1. First MTP joint applied anatomy. (*A*) Plantar structures as depicted from a dorsal view. (*B*) Collateral ligament view. (*From* Early JS. Fractures and dislocations of the midfoot and forefoot. In: Bucholz R, Heckman J, editors. Rockwood and Green's fractures in adults. 5th edition. Philadelphia: Lippincott Williams and Wilkins; 2001. p. 2229; with permission.)

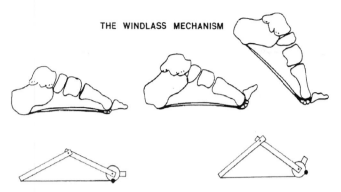

Fig. 2. The windlass mechanism and its effect on the midfoot. (*From* Mann RA, Schakel II ME. Surgical correction of rheumatoid forefoot deformities. Foot Ankle Int 1995;16:1–6; with permission. Copyright © 1995 by the American Orthopaedic Foot and Ankle Society (AOFAS).)

MTP fusion at an average of 26° of dorsiflexion did indeed exhibit a windlass-mechanistic effect, with a significant number of plantarflexed first rays. Patients who had rheumatoid arthritis were included [6].

Pathophysiology

The pathologic changes brought on by rheumatoid arthritis have been studied extensively. Through an autoimmune reaction, a severe synovitis extends to the bone, thereby destroying the articular cartilage and attenuating the capsuloligamentous–sesamoid complex. The once superior supporting structures are now incapable of stabilizing the joint under the large forces experienced on a daily basis.

The first MTP joint drifts into progressive valgus and rarely dorsal subluxation. The weightbearing function is then transferred to the lesser metatarsals. This occurs in the face of ongoing synovitis and destruction of the lesser toes, which begin to exhibit subluxation or frank dislocation. The plantar aponeurosis acts as a pulley in displacing the plantar fat pads distally along with the soft-tissue structures inserting onto the proximal phalanges. Without functional fat pads present beneath the MTP heads, intractable plantar callosities develop [7]. At least half of all patients who have rheumatoid arthritis experience collapse of the longitudinal arch [8], and this can arise from midfoot and from hindfoot synovitis [1].

The great toe has also been described to drift into a dorsiflexed position and even a hallux primus varus. Additionally, a pronation deformity of greater than 20° has been associated with severe hallux valgus. Both of these deformities can distribute additional force over the plantar-medial aspect of the foot, the aspect that bears a good deal of weight. Also, approximately 40% of patients who have rheumatoid arthritis may exhibit interphalangeal (IP) hyperextension with associated shoe discomfort [7].

Treatment

Nonoperative

The accepted initial treatment of rheumatoid forefoot dysfunction is conservative management. Drug therapy with nonsteroidal anti-inflammatory drugs used as first-line therapy and immunosuppressives used in late stages of the disease remains standard. Routine heel cord stretching may prove beneficial in ankle and subtalar joint involvement. Shoe inserts and modifications along with braces and crutches may also be implemented for symptomatic relief.

Operative

When conservative treatment fails to alleviate patients' symptoms, operative intervention is indicated. As described, the forefoot experiences joint destruction that alters the biomechanics of the entire foot. As such, the operative goal should then be to mitigate pain and restore the natural biomechanics of the forefoot.

A multitude of surgeries have been performed in the past to address the rheumatoid forefoot and the concurrent disability. Perhaps the most universally accepted of these methods involved resection arthroplasty of each MTP joint [9–14]. Although this surgery is standard of care for the lesser MTP joints, controversy existed with regard to the first MTP joint. In the short term, lateral metatarsal pressure is relieved and the lesser toes show good realignment. After time, however, common complications following this procedure include recurrent hallux valgus, plantar keratoses, and metatarsalgia [10,11,15–17]. Additionally Watson [15] showed that hallux support was lessened after resection.

Recently Grondal and colleagues [18] prospectively compared Mayo resection (resection of the first metatarsal head) of the first MTP joint to hallux MTP arthrodesis in 33 patients who had rheumatoid arthritis. It was their contention that the previous poor results were based on Keller-type resections that remove the proximal phalanx and the plantar plate, thus causing instability. The Mayo resection, in contrast, preserves the plantar structures and allows the first MTP to retain its flexion capacity. Additionally they contended that patients following resection were as or more satisfied with the procedure than with arthrodesis, regardless of cosmesis, balance, and weightbearing. After 3 years there was no statistically significant difference between the groups with regard to satisfaction, recurrence, or shoe wear, leading to a conclusion that Mayo resection may still be a valid option for patients with rheumatoid arthritis [18].

Mann and Thompson [19], however, found that following a resection arthroplasty procedure, hallux valgus did indeed recur, the toes tended to displace dorsally, and the fat pads again displaced distally. They added that during the end of the stance phase of gait, all toes were forced into dorsiflexion and lateral deviation, likely secondary to the destabilization of the MTP joints after the procedure [19].

Coughlin [20] describes the key factor in rheumatoid forefoot reconstruction as being the achievement of stable realignment of the first ray. With the previously noted complications of resection arthroplasty, hallux MTP arthrodesis offers a solution to first ray complications. Theoretically medial column weightbearing should be maintained, thus mitigating stress on the lesser metatarsals and maintaining a proper alignment of the corresponding fat pads [21]. Mann and Coughlin [7] describes first MTP joint arthrodesis in a patient who has rheumatoid arthritis as providing stability that permanently corrects the hallux deformity, permits ordinary shoe wear, and when combined with excisional arthroplasty of the lesser metatarsals, provides first MTP rigidity necessary in mitigating lesser metatarsal stress and maintaining proper fat pad alignment [7].

Harris-mat studies have shown in the past that indeed hallux MTP arthrodesis provides greater weightbearing capacity on the first metatarsal. Henry and Waugh [22] compared preoperative and postoperative weightbearing in patients treated with excisional arthroplasty versus those treated with hallux MTP fusion. They reported increased weightbearing in 80% of the arthrodesis group compared with 40% of the excisional group [22]. This report was substantiated by Mann and Thompson [19] and Coughlin [20], with 89% and 100%, respectively, demonstrating increased weightbearing capacity.

There are various techniques described in performing a hallux arthrodesis. Included are intramedullary Steinmann pins, crossed Kirschner wires, cerclage wires, staples, compression screws axially or obliquely placed, external compression clamps, external fixators, and dorsal compression plates with intra-articular fixation [23]. Additionally joint surface preparations vary also, including cartilage denuding, cone and socket preparation, planar cartilage removal (saw), and machined conical reaming [24–26]. Coughlin [20] reported a 100% fusion rate in long-term follow-up on 58 feet using a six-hole mini-compression plate and a cross-compression screw, with joint preparation involving cannulated cup-shaped reamers after resection of the proximal phalanx, metatarsal head, and medial eminence. This corroborated his earlier findings with regard to dorsal plate use for fusion, wherein a 100% fusion rate was attained in 35 feet [24]. An overall successful hallux MTP fusion rate has been reported to be greater than 90% [20].

Although hallux MTP fusion is successfully achieved in most patients, the optimal form of fixation continues to be explored. Several biomechanical studies on cadavers have reported results comparing first MTP fusion techniques and joint preparations. Sykes and Hughes [27] found crossed-cancellous screws and planar joint excision most stable, whereas Curtis and colleagues [28] showed conical reaming with an interfragmentary screw conferred the most stable arthrodesis. Rongstad and colleagues [29] compared cancellous screw with mini-plate fixation, Herbert screw, and

Steinmann pin fixation. The mini-plate/interfragmentary screw fixation and the Herbert screw provided the best fixation. Finally, Politi and colleagues [23] compared surface excision with interfragmentary screw, surface excision with crossed Kirschner wires, surface excision with a lag screw and dorsal mini-plate, surface excision and machined conical reaming with dorsal mini-plate and no lag screw, and planar surface excision with interfragmentary lag screw. Their report suggested that the most stable technique for obtaining fusion was the combination of an oblique lag screw and dorsal mini-plate [23]. This substantiates Rongstad's findings and seems to support the clinical studies using this type of fixation [20,24,29].

Hallux MTP sagittal alignment must also be taken into account when fusing the first MTP joint. Fusion in excessive valgus may result in a widened forefoot [20]. Successful hallux valgus angles postoperatively range from 15° to 30° [19,20,30,31]. Fitzgerald [30] reported the finding that symptomatic IP arthritis increases threefold when the hallux valgus fusion angle is less than 20°. This was not substantiated by Coughlin, however [20].

First MTP dorsiflexion angle also proves critical in patient outcome. Optimal MTP dorsiflexion angle after fusion has been reported between 15° and 40° [20,30–33]. Factors such as pes planus severity, tarsometatarsal hypermobility, and measurement point of reference have all influenced the recommended dorsiflexion angle. A theoretic optimal range is obtained by adding 5° to 15° of phalangeal dorsiflexion to the anatomic 15° of first metatarsal inclination [20]. The angle of inclination, or the angle in the lateral plane between the long axis of the first digit and the floor, may provide a more accurate measurement, because it constitutes the functional angle by which the patient walks (Fig. 3) [18]. A significantly higher rate of IP arthrosis has been reported when first MTP dorsiflexion is less than 20° [20]. The rate of IP arthritis after the first MTP fusion has been reported in the literature to be 30% to 67% [11,19,20,32]. Although threaded Steinmann pin fixation may influence the progression of IP arthritis, a clinical significance is not present [32]. Additionally patient shoe preference must be taken into account, because high-heeled shoes may require an increased dorsiflexion angle. Dorsiflexion angles less than 10° and greater than 40° have influenced shoe wear also [33,34].

Finally, rotation of the hallux must be addressed when performing a hallux MTP arthrodesis. Hand-held conical reamers have been implemented in

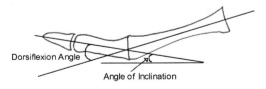

Fig. 3. Angle of inclination (*AI*) and dorsiflexion angle (*DFA*) represent two methods used in measuring the amount of dorsiflexion in first MTP joint arthrodesis.

the past [30,31,33,35], with an overall fusion rate for these reamers reportedly attaining 92% [24]. Metatarsal head orientation with regard to dorsiflexion and valgus, however, is determined by the reamer, thus precluding any further adjustment. In an attempt to counteract this shortcoming, Coughlin [24] helped develop a cup-shaped cannulated reamer that accepted a 0.062 Kirschner wire. In doing so, stability while reaming is maintained and congruous female and male surfaces are created. Hallux MTP dorsiflexion, varus/valgus alignment, and rotation are easily aligned for arthrodesis [24]. A final neutral rotational alignment of the hallux is optimal (Fig. 4) [24,36,37].

Arthrodesis as a salvage procedure

With regard to rheumatoid arthritis, treatment failures of the hallux MTP are not uncommon. As described, first metatarsal head excision may lead to hallux valgus, plantar keratoses, and metatarsalgia. Trnka [17] describes first MTP fusion with lesser metatarsal shortening osteotomies as viable salvage to failed resection. Additionally, silicone implants have been described as a means of restoring rheumatoid first MTP joint motion [38]. High rates of implant failure and silicone synovitis, however, have all but led to its abandonment [39,40]. When combined with bone grafting, first MTP fusion has shown good results as a salvage procedure for failed silicone arthroplasty [41].

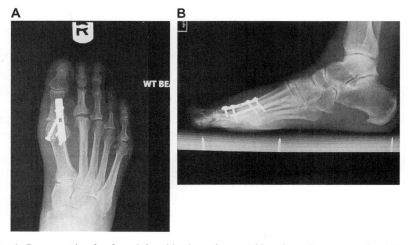

Fig. 4. Postoperative forefoot deformities in a rheumatoid patient. Anteroposterior (A) and lateral (B) radiographs demonstrating the hallux MTP fusion with a dorsal mini-plate with interfragmentary screw fixation.

Complications

The rate of complications following hallux MTP fusion in patients who have rheumatoid arthritis varies depending on such factors as type of fixation, patient selection, and operative technique. Failure of compression screw fixation is rare [42]. Nonunion is uncommon also and may result in an acceptable pseudarthroses [24,35]. An overall failure rate ranges from 10% to 23% [24,33,43]. Albert and Wapner [44] describes metatarsal shaft fractures secondary to stress risers caused by Steinmann pin removal, and he cautions similar outcomes after dorsal mini-plate removal. Interphalangeal arthrosis, perhaps the most common complication, is described.

Summary

First MTP joint fusion provides a permanent medial support that serves to prevent further deformity of the lesser toes of a patient who has rheumatoid arthritis. The anatomy and biomechanics of the hallux MTP joint are complex, thus making proper operative arthrodesis of paramount importance. Fixation type, sagittal alignment, varus/valgus alignment, rotation, and joint surface preparation all represent critical factors to consider before fusion. Arthrodesis of the hallux MTP joint in a patient who has rheumatoid arthritis is a highly successful procedure with low complication rates that produces a stable foot and improves quality of life.

References

[1] Weinfeld S, Schon L. Hallux metatarsophalangeal arthritis. Clin Orthop Relat Res 1998;349: 9–19.

[2] Johnson R, Buck P. Total replacement arthroplasty of the first metatarsophalangeal joint. Foot Ankle 1981;1:307–14.

[3] Hansen S Jr. Functional reconstruction of the foot and ankle. Philadelphia: Lippincott Williams & Wilkins; 2000.

[4] Maskill J, Anderson J, Bohay D. First ray injuries. Foot Ankle Clin 2006;11(1):143–63.

[5] Hicks J. The mechanics of the foot. II: The plantar aponeurosis and the arch. J Anat 1954;66: 812–4.

[6] Lombardi C, Silhanek A, Connolly F, et al. The effect of first metatarsophalangeal joint arthrodesis on the first ray and the medial longitudinal arch: a radiographic study. J Foot Ankle Surg 2002;41(2):96–103.

[7] Mann RA, Coughlin MJ. Surgery of the foot and ankle. 6th edition. St. Louis (MO): Mosby Inc.; 1993.

[8] Spiegel TM, Spiegel JS. Rheumatoid arthritis in the foot and ankle: diagnosis, pathology, and treatment: the relationship between foot and ankle deformity and disease duration in 50 patients. Foot Ankle 1982;2:318–24.

[9] Goldie L, Bremell T, Althoff B, et al. Metatarsal head resection in the treatment of the rheumatoid forefoot. Scand J Rheumatol 1983;12:106–12.

[10] McGarvey SR, Johnson KA. Keller arthroplasty in combination with resection arthroplasty of the lesser metatarsophalangeal joints in rheumatoid arthritis. Foot Ankle 1988;9:75–80.

[11] Vahvanen V, Piirainen H, Kettunen P. Resection arthroplasty in rheumatoid arthritis: a follow-up study of 100 patients. Scand J Rheumatol 1980;9:257–65.

[12] van der Heiden KW, Rasker JJ, Jacobs JW. Kates forefoot arthroplasty in rheumatoid arthritis. J Rheumotol 1992;19:1545–50.

[13] Craxford AD, Stevens J, Park C. Management of the deformed rheumatoid forefoot: a comparison of surgical and conservative methods. Clin Orthop Rel Res 1982;166:121–6.

[14] Raunio P, Lehtimaki M, Eerola M, et al. Resection arthroplasty versus arthrodesis of the first metatarsophalangeal joint for hallux valgus in rheumatoid arthritis. Clin Orthop Rel Res 1987;11:173–8.

[15] Watson MS. A long term follow-up of forefoot arthroplasty. J Bone Joint Surg 1974;56: 527–33.

[16] Hasselo LG, Willkens RF, Toomey HE, et al. Forefoot surgery in rheumatoid arthritis: subjective assessment of outcome. Foot Ankle 1987;8:148–51.

[17] Trnka HJ. Arthrodesis procedures for the salvage of the hallux metatarsophalangeal joint. Foot Ankle Clin 2000;5(3):673–86.

[18] Grondal L, Hedstrom M, Stark A. Arthrodesis compared to Mayo resection of the first metatarsophalangeal joint in total rheumatoid forefoot reconstruction. Foot Ankle Int 2005;26(2):135–9.

[19] Mann RA, Thompson FM. Arthrodesis of the first metatarsophalangeal joint for hallux valgus in rheumatoid arthritis. J Bone Joint Surg Am 1984;66(5):687–92.

[20] Coughlin MJ. Rheumatoid forefoot reconstruction. J Bone Joint Surg Am 2000;82(3): 322–41.

[21] Mulcahy D, Daniels TR, Lau JT, et al. Rheumatoid forefoot deformity: a comparison study of 2 functional methods of reconstruction. J Rheumatol 2003;30:1440–50.

[22] Henry APJ, Waugh W. The use of footprints in assessing the results of operations for hallux valgus: a comparison of Keller's operation and arthrodesis. J Bone Joint Surg Am 1975; 57(4):478–81.

[23] Politi J, Hayes J, Njus G, et al. First metatarsal-phalangeal joint arthrodesis: a biomechanical assessment of stability. Foot Ankle Int 2003;24(4):332–7.

[24] Coughlin MJ. Arthrodesis of the first metatarsophalangeal joint with mini-fragment plate fixation. Orthopedics 1990;13:1037–44.

[25] Coughlin MJ. Arthrodesis of the first metatarsophalangeal joint. Orthop Rev 1990;19: 177–86.

[26] Johansson JE, Barrington TW. Con arthrodesis of the first metatarsophalangeal joint. Foot Ankle 1984;4(5):244–8.

[27] Sykes A, Hughes AW. A biomechanical study using cadaveric toes to test the stability of fixation techniques employed in arthrodesis of the first metatarsophalangeal joint. Foot Ankle Int 1986;7:18–25.

[28] Curtis MJ, Myerson M, Jinnah RH, et al. Arthrodesis of the first metatarsophalangeal joint: a biomechanical study of internal fixation techniques. Foot Ankle Int 1993;14:395–9.

[29] Rongstad KM, Miller GJ, Vander Griend RA, et al. A biomechanical comparison of four fixation methods of first metatarsophalangeal joint arthrodesis. Foot Ankle Int 1994;15: 415–9.

[30] Fitzgerald JAW. A review of long-term results of arthrodesis of the first metatarsophalangeal joint. J Bone Joint Surg Am 1969;51(3):488–93.

[31] Raymakers R, Waugh W. The treatment of metatarsalgia with hallux valgus. J Bone Joint Surg Am 1971;53(4):684–7.

[32] Mann RA, Schakel ME II. Surgical correction of rheumatoid forefoot deformities. Foot Ankle Int 1995;16:1–6.

[33] Moynihan FJ. Arthrodesis of the metatarsophalangeal joint of the great toe. J Bone Joint Surg Am 1967;49(3):544–51.

[34] Beauchamp CG, Kirby T, Rudge SR, et al. Fusion of the first metatarsophalangeal joint in forefoot arthroplasty. Clin Orthop Relat Res 1984;190:249–53.

[35] McKeever DC. Arthrodesis of the first metatarsophalangeal joint of the big toe for hallux valgus and hallux rigidus. J Bone Joint Surg Am 1952;34:129–34.

[36] Lipscombe PR. Arthrodesis of the first metatarsophalangeal joint for severe bunions and hallux rigidus. Clin Orthop Relat Res 1979;142:48–54.

[37] Harrison MHM, Harvey FJ. Arthrodesis of the first metatarsophalangeal joint for hallux valgus and hallux rigidus. J Bone Joint Surg Am 1963;45:471–80.

[38] Hanyu T, Yamazuki H, Ishikawa H, et al. Flexible hinge toe implant arthroplasty for rheumatoid arthritis of the first metatarsophalangeal joint: long-term results. J Orthop Sci 2001;6:141–7.

[39] Gordon M, Bullough PG. Synovial and osseous inflammation in failed silicone-rubber prostheses. J Bone Joint Surg Am 1982;64:574–80.

[40] Worsing RA Jr, Engber WD, Lange TA. Reactive synovitis from particulate silastic. J Bone Joint Surg Am 1982;64:581–5.

[41] Hecht PJ, Gibbons MJ, Wapner KL, et al. Arthrodesis of the first metatarsophalangeal joint to salvage failed silicone implant arthroplasty. Foot Ankle Int 1997;18:383–90.

[42] Riggs SA, Johnson EW. McKeever arthrodesis for the painful hallux. Foot Ankle 1983;3(5): 248–53.

[43] Gimple K, Anspacher JC, Kopta JA. Metatarsophalangeal joint fusion of the great toe. Orthopedics 1978;1(6):462–7.

[44] Albert TJ, Wapner KL. Metatarsal shaft fracture after first metatarsophalangeal joint fusion: a complication of Steinmann pin fixation. Foot Ankle 1993;14(2):107–10.

ELSEVIER
SAUNDERS

Foot Ankle Clin N Am
12 (2007) 405–416

FOOT AND
ANKLE CLINICS

Hallux Metatarsophalangeal Arthroplasty in the Rheumatoid Forefoot

C. Senthil Kumar, FRCS(Tr&Orth)[a],*,
G. Holt, MRCS[b]

[a]Department of Orthopaedic and Trauma Surgery, Glasgow Royal Infirmary,
84 Castle Street, Glasgow, G4 0SF, UK
[b]Department of Orthopaedic and Trauma Surgery, West of Scotland Deanery,
Glasgow Royal Infirmary, 84 Castle Street, Glasgow, G4 0SF, UK

Rheumatoid disease is a systemic inflammatory disorder characterized by a symmetric polyarthritis that typically affects the neck, shoulder, elbow, wrist, hands, and feet. Approximately 20% of patients who have rheumatoid arthritis present initially with foot and ankle symptoms. The prevalence of forefoot deformities in adults who have chronic rheumatoid disease is approximately 90% [1]. Both feet are normally affected, although the resulting deformities may not be symmetric [1]. Chronic synovial inflammation leads to capsular distention, articular cartilage destruction, subchondral bone erosion, and a loss of collateral ligament integrity. The resulting soft-tissue instability leads to the common rheumatoid forefoot deformities. The typical rheumatoid forefoot is characterized by hallux valgus, plantar displacement of the metatarsal heads, and a varus position of the little toe. Subluxation or dislocation of the proximal phalanges dorsally on the metatarsal heads results in migration of the plantar fat pad distally beneath the hyperextended toes. This leads to the formation of large painful callosities and bursae under the metatarsal heads. The intrinsic–extrinsic muscle balance is lost and fixed clawing of the lesser toes develops, resulting in painful, thickened calluses dorsally over the proximal interphalangeal joints and medially over the first metatarsal head. Deformities of the forefoot may also be caused by arthritis and deformity of the hindfoot.

---

* Corresponding author.
E-mail address: senthil.kumar@northglasgow.scot.nhs.uk (C. Senthil Kumar).

1083-7515/07/$ - see front matter © 2007 Elsevier Inc. All rights reserved.
doi:10.1016/j.fcl.2007.04.001

Conservative treatment remains the mainstay of early management of rheumatoid arthritis with disease modifying pharmacologic therapy to slow progression of the disease. Other interventions include physical therapy and steroid injections. Shoe modifications and ambulatory aids are frequently beneficial. Despite such measures, some patients continue to deteriorate and surgical correction may be indicated. The surgical correction of the rheumatoid forefoot is directed at stable realignment, reduced pain, improved mobility, reduced pressure, and easier fitting of a shoe. The concepts and principles of reconstruction of the forefoot have been subject to modification over time. Several operative procedures designed to correct components of the rheumatoid forefoot have been described. Methods for the treatment of a symptomatic hallux valgus deformity have included resection of the first metatarsal head [2–7], arthrodesis of the first metatarsophalangeal (MTP) joint [8–13], excision of the proximal phalanx (Keller's operation) [2,3,6,14], and silicone hinge replacement [15–18]. The ideal surgical treatment for the hallux in the rheumatoid forefoot, however, remains controversial. Outcome studies are often limited by the duration of follow-up, small study populations, failure to document radiographic outcome, and a lack of comparable, validated objective postoperative assessment. In this article, the authors discuss the surgical treatment options and reported outcomes for arthroplasty of the first MTP (MTP1) joint in the rheumatoid forefoot.

Resection arthroplasty of the first metatarsal head

Resection arthroplasty of the first metatarsal head is well documented as part of forefoot reconstruction in the rheumatoid foot [2–7,19,20]. Hoffman [19] is credited with the first description of this technique in 1912 when he resected all five metatarsal heads through a single transverse plantar incision. Subsequently several modifications to this technique have been reported, including dorsal/plantar incisions, repositioning the plantar fat pad, and combinations of excision of the metatarsal heads and excision of the proximal aspect of the proximal phalanges [2–7,19,20].

Barton [3] described the results of 65 operations performed with various techniques, including resection of the first metatarsal head and resection of the base of the proximal phalanx without arthrodesis. Although most patients were satisfied because they had received some relief from pain, only 29 (45%) were pain-free. Stockley and colleagues [21] reported that 42 (70%) of 60 feet were pain-free at 3 years following a plantar incision with resection of all metatarsal heads and replacement of the fat pad. Patsalis and colleagues [22] followed 36 feet in 23 patients for an average of more than 10 years after resection of all five metatarsal heads through a plantar incision and found a 56% rate of dissatisfaction because of pain. Other investigators have found less than satisfactory results with resection arthroplasty of the first MTP joint.

Van der Heijen and colleagues [23] reported the results of Kate's forefoot arthroplasty in 74 feet of 41 patients who had rheumatoid arthritis after a mean follow-up of 5.2 years. Outcome was considered to be good by 38 patients and poor by 3 patients. The average walking distance had doubled. The mean hallux valgus angle was reduced from 46° to 27°. Surgical results seemed to depend on the quality of the arc of the remaining stumps. Re-operations were necessary in 16 feet of 10 patients because of too prominent distal metatarsal stumps. Despite the absence of pain, 28 patients were not satisfied with the function of the hallux.

Keller's procedure

The assessment of outcome after resection arthroplasty is somewhat complicated by the combination of techniques termed "resection arthroplasty," which often include excision of the proximal phalanx. Studies have shown that removal of part or a significant portion of the proximal phalanx results in a substantial reduction of the weightbearing function of the hallux, resulting in callosities under the lesser metatarsals caused by transfer lesions [14].

Furhmann and Anders [24] performed a retrospective study of 188 patients (254 feet) who had rheumatoid arthritis and compared the late results of Keller's procedure with those of first metatarsal head excision by Hueter-Mayo technique after 7.9 years. More than 60% of the Keller group and 30% of the Hueter-Mayo group were suffering from persistent metatarsalgia caused by increased forefoot pressure and were experiencing pain around the great toe. Plantar callosities, recurrent hallux valgus deformity, lack of plantar flexion, and weakened push-off were more frequent after Keller's procedure.

McGarvey and Johnston [25] reviewed the results of the Keller arthroplasty in 29 patients (49 feet) in combination with resection arthroplasty of the forefoot in patients who had rheumatoid arthritis. The average age of the patients was 55.4 years, and the average follow-up period was 4.9 years. All feet had resection of the metatarsal heads and base of the proximal phalanges of the lesser toes and a Keller arthroplasty of the MTP1 joint. The results were satisfactory in 16 feet, satisfactory with some reservations in 21 feet, satisfactory with major reservations in 7 feet, and unsatisfactory in 5 feet. For 40 of the 49 feet (82%), the patients stated that they would repeat the procedure knowing the results achieved. The major causes of patient reservations and lack of satisfaction were return of the hallux valgus deformity and pain (53%), forefoot instability (27%), and continuing metatarsalgia (20%). The investigators concluded that Keller resection arthroplasty of the MTP1 joint results in an increased number of unsatisfactory results attributable to recurrent pain and deformity of the MTP joint.

There is a concern that excision of the hallux MTP joint may result in increased load bearing by the lesser metatarsals. A high level of recurrent hallux valgus, metatarsalgia, and recurrent plantar keratosis has been reported after long-term follow-up. The prevalence of recurrent hallux valgus or subtotal correction after resection arthroplasty has been reported to be as high as 53% to 68% in some of the largest series [23,25–27]. Recurrent plantar keratoses have been reported to occur, with the prevalence ranging from 36% to 61% following resection arthroplasty of the MTP1 joint [23,25–27].

Resection arthroplasty of the lesser MTP joints may weaken support for the hallux [28]. Maintenance of the alignment of the first MTP joint with arthrodesis protects not only the hallux but also the lesser MTP joints from recurrent deformity [11]. With an unstable MTP1 joint following excisional arthroplasty, lateral pressure from the hallux may cause lateral deviation or malalignment of the lesser MTP joints [26]. This may lead to a deterioration of outcome in time with recurrent deformity and metatarsalgia [6,25,26,29]. Pedobarographic studies of the distribution of plantar pressure after resection arthroplasty have reported reduced or absent pressure across the toes with the transmission of the weightbearing load to the end of the resected metatarsals with nearly identical pressures exerted at the lesser toes and the first ray [14]. Such findings are more marked when the base of the proximal phalanx is excised [14]. The result is a relative overload of the lesser metatarsal heads, which may lead to metatarsalgia and plantar keratosis [16,30,31]. Henry and Waugh [14] evaluated postoperative weightbearing in a study of 170 feet, half of which had been treated with excisional arthroplasty and half of which had been treated with MTP arthrodesis. Substantial weightbearing on the first ray was noted in 80% of feet that had been treated with MTP arthrodesis compared with only 40% of feet that had been treated with excisional arthroplasty.

These findings aside, arthrodesis of the MTP1 joint for rheumatoid forefoot deformity is not always possible. Bone loss secondary to subchondral erosions and osteoporosis may mean that from a technical point of view rigid fixation is difficult if not impossible. Similarly, patient characteristics may be such that performing a more technically challenging procedure that relies on bony union for success may not be desirable. Outcomes in patients who fail to unite have been reported as highly unsatisfactory compared with excision arthroplasty [32]. Thomas and colleagues [20] reported the results of 37 forefoot arthroplasties in 20 patients who were reviewed at an average of 5.5 years. The procedure involved excision of all five metatarsal heads through three dorsal incisions. All of the patients in the study were satisfied with the results of the operation at follow-up and no revision surgeries were undertaken during the period of the study.

Arthrodesis versus resection arthroplasty

Several studies have compared patient outcomes of arthrodesis and resection arthroplasty of the MTP1 joint. There is little in the way of high quality evidence to scientifically evaluate the compared outcomes of these two procedures. Grondal and colleagues [33] reported the only prospective, randomized study to date. In this series 31 patients were allocated to either arthrodesis or Mayo resection of the first MTP joint as part of a reconstruction of the rheumatoid forefoot. Twenty-nine patients were re-examined after a mean of 72 months (57–80 months). Excellent patient satisfaction was reported with a significant, lasting reduction of the foot function index. No statistically significant difference was observed between the groups. There were no significant differences in recurrence of the deformity, the need for special shoes, gait velocity, step length, plantar moment, mean pressure, or the position of the center of force under the forefoot. This study is limited in the conclusions that may be drawn, however, by low statistical power as a consequence of small patient numbers. Several other studies have investigated outcomes between these procedures; however, they are either retrospective or lack patient randomization.

Mulcahy and colleagues [34] compared the results of two different forefoot procedures, presenting a stable first ray (52 feet) and resection arthroplasty (86 feet). The resection group had a significantly longer follow-up (102 versus 36 months) and was older, but no differences in the SF-36, foot function index, and Western Ontario and McMaster Osteoarthritis Index (WOMAC) scores were observed. The stable group had a significantly increased walking distance, higher satisfaction with cosmetic result, less pain from the foot, and fewer plantar calluses. Patients were followed pedobarographically with a more favorable outcome for the stable group with a physiologically greater distribution of weightbearing forces through the first and lesser toes. This study, however, has several methodologic flaws in that it is retrospective, patients are not matched, some of the patients in the stable group had no surgery, and the follow-up times are significantly different between cohorts.

Huges and colleagues [32] studied 34 painful, deformed rheumatoid feet treated by excision of all five metatarsal heads compared with 34 similar feet in which the lesser metatarsal heads were excised and the first MTP joint was arthrodesed. In the latter group, one third had failure of fusion of the hallux, and this produced the worst results. Metatarsalgia and plantar callosities were more common after excision arthroplasty, but shoe fitting and correction of deformity were better in this group. The results were more variable in the fusion group, and the complication and re-operation rates were higher.

Beauchamp and colleagues [35] reported the results in 37 patients with 64 arthroplasty operations (34 with fusion and 30 with excision of the first joint). Fusion produced a better cosmetic appearance of the foot, facilitated fitting with normal shoes, and improved overall balance. Pedobarographic measurements during gait indicated that more weight was transmitted through the medial ray when the first MTP joint was fused. Residual pain in the foot was often caused by irregular trimming of the metatarsals. There was no difference in relief of pain between fused and unfused patients. Radiologic degeneration of the interphalangeal joint of the great toe was more common following fusion, and the investigators concluded fusion was inadvisable if there was pre-existing disease in the interphalangeal joint.

Vahvanen and colleagues [26] reported the follow-up results 1 to 11 years (mean, 5 years) after resection arthroplasty of the forefoot or arthrodesis of the first MTP joint performed on 100 patients (179 feet) with rheumatoid arthritis. Resection arthroplasty of the lesser toes was performed from the plantar approach in 167 feet. The Keller or Mayo operation was performed on the MTP1 joint in 129 feet. Arthrodesis of the MTP1 joint was done in 17 feet. According to the subjective assessment, results after surgery were considered good by 49 patients (91 feet, 51%), fair by 44 (76 feet, 42%), and poor by 7 (12 feet, 7%). These seven patients complained of persistent pain or a disabling deformity of the toes, or both. Although these results were generally satisfactory, the objective results were not good. At follow-up more than 50% of the patients had recidivistic callosities, a hallux valgus deformity, a dorsal dislocation and lateral deviation of the lesser toes, or radiologically observable bony proliferations of the distal ends of the metatarsals or a combination of these. All patients in whom a proximal interphalangeal joint of the hallux was surgically or spontaneously fused were satisfied: the stiff joint was painless on walking. The investigators concluded that when destruction of the MTP1 joint is severe and painful, arthrodesis is recommended.

Vandeputte and colleagues [36] compared the subjective, clinical, and pedodynographic results of two groups of patients undergoing reconstructive surgery for rheumatoid forefoot deformities. Thirty-eight patients (59 feet) underwent a Keller arthroplasty of the MTP1 joint and a Hoffmann resection of the lesser metatarsal heads. The mean follow-up was 35 months. Forty-eight patients (62 feet) underwent an arthrodesis of the MTP1 joint and Hoffmann resection of the lesser metatarsal heads. The mean follow-up was 25 months. In 10 feet the arthrodesis was performed as a revision procedure of a failed Keller arthroplasty. Better load-bearing of the first ray with relative unloading of the central metatarsal heads was noted in the arthrodesis group. Subjective evaluation of the procedure was slightly better in the Keller group. Ninety-three percent of the patients in the Keller group were satisfied or satisfied with minor reservations, versus 87% in the arthrodesis group however, this was not statistically significant. Recurrent deformity was not more prominent in the Keller group; however, it was concluded that follow-up time may not have been sufficient to make any conclusions on long-term outcome.

Silicone implant arthroplasty

Silicone interposition arthroplasty of the MTP1 joint has been reported as an alternative to arthrodesis or resection arthroplasty in the rheumatoid forefoot. The silicone stemmed implant to replace the base of the proximal phalanx was developed in 1967 to provide an alternative treatment for hallux valgus and hallux rigidus. Silicone elastomer was introduced in 1974, which was designed to be more resistant to tear propagation than its precursor [37]. These hinged prostheses acted as spacers, allowing more flexibility compared with an arthrodesis and improved stability compared with a resection arthroplasty [37]. Early results of silastic joint replacement of the MTP1 joint were encouraging [37,38]. Patients reported a reduction in pain, had good functional results, and often had no restriction in footwear. The hinged silicone prosthesis was initially believed to be durable and biocompatible. During the early 1980s, however, reports of premature wear and silicone synovitis began to appear in the literature [39–43]. Although the implant itself is inert, abrasion of the implants was found to produce microscopic particles that caused an inflammatory synovitis. Implant wear was also found to cause a silicone particulate lymphadenitis and cystic osteolysis in cancellous bone adjacent to the implants [44–55]. Titanium grommets were added to the procedure to protect the soft implant from bone abrasion leading to particularization [45,56,57].

Bommireddy and colleagues [15] reviewed outcomes in 32 patients (42 feet) with double-stem silicone implant arthroplasty of the MTP1 joint reviewed at an average of 8 years (range, 4–19 years) in patients who had hallux valgus and osteoarthritis. Twenty-eight of the 32 patients were very satisfied with the procedure. No patients were dissatisfied. Pain relief was subjectively excellent or good in 28 patients. Radiographs showed sclerosis around all prostheses. Cysts with bony erosions were noted in 17 cases. Twelve had clinical features of silicone synovitis in the early postoperative period, but this was not present at final review despite radiologic findings of new bone formation (57%) and localized osteolysis (40%). No patient required revision surgery. Patients were found to have very good subjective and objective results despite poor radiologic results. As such, the investigators suggested a role for double-stemmed silicone implant arthroplasty in low-demand patients.

Hanyu and colleagues [16] report the results of silicone hinge interposition arthroplasty of the MTP1 joint, combined with a shortening oblique osteotomy of the metatarsal neck in the lesser toes in patients who have rheumatoid arthritis. Follow-up information was available for 60 feet in 39 patients who had an average follow-up of 12 years. Twenty-nine patients (74%) were satisfied with the outcome after surgery, 7 were satisfied but had some pain or recurrent deformities, and 3 were unsatisfied. Radiologically visible fracture was identified in nine implants. Four implants were removed because of infection (n = 2) or recurrent deformity (n = 2) and no implant was removed secondary to silicone synovitis. With revision as the endpoint, the implant survival rate was 93% at 10 years, and with radiographic implant fracture as the endpoint, the implant survival rate was 87% at 10 years.

Cracchiolo and colleagues [17] reported on 86 implants with an average 6.8-year follow-up. Forty-nine (57%) were in 32 patients who had rheumatoid arthritis who also had resection of the lateral metatarsal heads. At an average 68.5 months follow-up, 84% of patients were satisfied completely, 13% were somewhat satisfied, and only 3% were dissatisfied. There were four (8%) implant failures for which the patients required revision surgery. Two were in patients who had rheumatoid arthritis.

Moeckle and colleagues [58] reported the outcomes of 67 implants in 45 patients who had rheumatoid arthritis with an average 6-year follow-up. All patients had excision of the lesser metatarsal heads, and an osteotomy of the base of the first metatarsal was performed in six feet. Eighty-seven percent of patients had good or excellent results. Of the nine (13%) feet with fair or poor results, six were attributable to insufficient resection of the lesser metatarsal heads. The remaining three (4%) were complications related to the implant and required implant removal resulting in a resection arthroplasty. Two were late infections and one was an implant fracture and dislocation 6 months after the index procedure. Overall there were two (3%) implant fractures and five (7%) implants with fragmentation, which were all asymptomatic.

Titanium grommets have been used in an attempt to increase the life of the silicone implant and protect it from fracture. Sebold and Cracchiolo [59] reported on 19 patients (25 feet) who had rheumatoid arthritis who all had silicone implants with titanium grommets. These patients were followed for an average of 51 months. The comparison group consisted of 19 patients (29 feet) who had rheumatoid arthritis who had silicone implants without grommets. These patients were followed for an average of 58 months. After radiographic analysis, there was significantly less evidence of radiolucency seen around implants protected by grommets. Clinical results between the two groups were not significantly different.

Swanson and colleagues [60] reported on the use of grommets in double-stem implants in 90 feet in 76 patients, of which 66 feet were in patients who had rheumatoid arthritis. At an average of 38 months follow-up, there was no evidence of silicone synovitis, bone resorption, grommet fracture, or implant fracture. There were three complications, all of which occurred in patients who had rheumatoid arthritis. Two of these complications were associated with deficient bone stock in patients who had revision surgery that resulted in rotation of the grommets and the implants. Clinically there was no difference in motion postoperatively compared with a previously reported group that did not receive grommets.

Rahman and Fagg [18] reported outcomes in 55 patients (78 feet) who had undergone silicone hemiarthroplasty for hallux valgus and hallux rigidus. Significant radiolucency was noted in 72% of all cases and around every prosthesis that had been implanted for longer than 4 years. The histologic findings in the three patients from whom the prosthesis was removed suggest that these radiologic changes indicate the presence of silicone granulomata. As in other series, a reasonable level of patient satisfaction was reported. The investigators, however, recommended that this procedure be abandoned.

Complications associated with silicone interposition arthroplasty include: a soft tissue inflammatory reaction (simulating infection), silicone particulate synovitis, osteolysis, prosthetic wear, dislocation, fragmentation, and silicone particle lymphadenitis [44–55]. The reported incidence of silicone synovitis is variable at between 0% and 26%; however, it does not always necessitate removal of the implant [15,17,51,61]. The incidence of implant fracture has been reported at between 1% and 8% [38,62]. Implant fracture is not necessarily associated with a poor outcome [59]. The implant functions mainly as a spacer, and if it remains intact long enough, fibrous tissue forms around the joint. This fibrous tissue then dictates the biomechanics of the joint, providing pain relief regardless of the condition of the implant [63].

Patient satisfaction scores after silastic interposition arthroplasty are favorable. Clinical outcomes reported by patients are better than one would expect from radiologic assessments. Results of several surgeons report high patient satisfaction scores in more than 84% of patients [38,61,63]. Many surgeons in the United Kingdom would be reluctant to use these implants in young, active patients who have hallux rigidus or hallux valgus because of risk for silicone synovitis, osteolysis, and lymphadenitis. In the low-demand elderly rheumatoid patient, these implants remain a potential treatment option.

Summary

Many procedures have been described for the treatment of hallux valgus and the related forefoot deformities associated with rheumatoid arthritis. Perhaps the most controversial issue has been the treatment of the first ray. Arthrodesis and resection are the two major surgical options for the MTP1 joint in reconstruction of the rheumatoid forefoot. In the literature the good to excellent success rates for resection vary from 51% to 93% [6,7,20,22,23]. The major complaints have been the high recurrence of hallux valgus, metatarsalgia, and plantar callosities, up to 53%, 36%, and 61%, respectively [23,25–27].

Arthrodesis of the MTP1 joint corrects malalignment of the first ray and creates a permanent angular correction that provides stability to the first ray, increases weightbearing on the first ray, and protects the lesser MTP joints from re-deformation. Decreased weightbearing on the lateral MTP joints diminishes the development of recurrent intractable plantar keratosis. Neither procedure is ideal, however, and results after MTP1 arthroplasty are not as good as those for other joints in the lower limb. The operative technique for arthrodesis is more demanding and involves a longer operating time. Proper alignment of the hallux is important and is fundamental to the success of the procedure but can be difficult to achieve. Interphalangeal joint degeneration is common although rarely symptomatic [11]. The rate of union is reported at 90% or more; however, results in patients who develop a nonunion are frequently less satisfactory [32].

Although arthrodesis generally has better reported results in recurrence of the deformity, reduced pressure under the lesser metatarsals, improved cosmesis, and reduced incidence of recurrent callosities, it is difficult to draw definite conclusions about how arthrodesis and resection arthroplasty compare. There has been only one prospective randomized controlled trial to date. This trial showed no obvious difference in outcome; however, it is limited in the conclusions that may be drawn because of low statistical power as a consequence of small patient numbers. Other comparative studies are either retrospective or not randomized. Additionally there is a lack of studies in which validated outcome scales were used, so comparison between studies has limited value. The polyarthritic nature of rheumatoid arthritis and its variable systemic and psychologic effects also makes valid comparisons in this patient group difficult [64].

Patients who present with forefoot deformity as a consequence of rheumatoid arthritis have varying degrees of pain, deformity, mobility, and expectation. No single procedure is suitable for every patient one is likely to encounter and fusion and some form of arthroplasty of the MTP1 joint have a place in the management of the rheumatoid forefoot. It is the role of the surgeon to decide which procedure is most appropriate for each individual case to obtain the most satisfactory results when treating this challenging surgical problem.

References

[1] Vainio K. Rheumatoid foot. Clinical study with pathological and roentgenological comments. Ann Chir Gynaecol Fenn 1956;45:1–107.

[2] Amuso SJ, Wissinger HA, Margolis HM, et al. Metatarsal head resection in the treatment of rheumatoid arthritis. Clin Orthop 1971;74:94–100.

[3] Barton NJ. Arthroplasty of the forefoot in rheumatoid arthritis. J Bone Joint Surg [Br] 1973; 55(1):126–33.

[4] Clayton ML. Surgery of the forefoot in rheumatoid arthritis. Clin Orthop 1960;16:136–40.

[5] Clayton ML. Surgery of the lower extremity in rheumatoid arthritis. J Bone Joint Surg [Am] 1963;45:1517–36.

[6] Craxford AD, Stevens J, Park C. Management of the deformed rheumatoid forefoot. A comparison of conservative and surgical methods. Clin Orthop 1982;166:121–6.

[7] Marmor L. Resection of the forefoot in rheumatoid arthritis. Clin Orthop 1975;108:223–7.

[8] MacClean CR, Silver WA. Dwyer's operation for the rheumatoid forefoot. Foot Ankle 1981;1:343–7.

[9] Mann RA, Thompson FM. Arthrodesis of the first metatarsophalangeal joint for hallux valgus in rheumatoid arthritis. J Bone Joint Surg [Am] 1984;66:687–92.

[10] Mann RA, Schakel ME II. Surgical correction of rheumatoid forefoot deformities. Foot Ankle Int 1995;16:1–6.

[11] Coughlin MJ. Rheumatoid forefoot reconstruction. A long-term follow-up study. J Bone Joint Surg [Am] 2000;82(3):322–41.

[12] Smith RW, Joanis TL, Maxwell PD. Great toe metatarsophalangeal joint arthrodesis: a user-friendly technique. Foot Ankle 1992;13(7):367–77.

[13] Coughlin MJ. Arthrodesis of the first metatarsophalangeal joint. Orthop Rev 1990;19:177–86.

[14] Henry APJ, Waugh W. The use of footprints in assessing the results of operations for hallux valgus. A comparison of Keller's operation and arthrodesis. J Bone Joint Surg [Br] 1975; 57(4):478–81.

[15] Bommireddy R, Singh SK, Sharma P, et al. Long-term follow-up of silastic joint replacement of the first metatarsophalangeal joint. The Foot 2003;13(3):151–5.

[16] Hanyu T, Yamazaki H, Ishikawa H, et al. Flexible hinge toe implant arthroplasty for rheumatoid arthritis of the first metatarsophalangeal joint: long-term results. J Orthop Sci 2001; 6(2):141–7.
[17] Cracchiolo A, Weltmer J, Lian G. Arthroplasty of the first metatarsophalangeal joint with double-stem silicone implant. J Bone Joint Surg [Am] 1992;74:552–63.
[18] Rahman H, Fagg PS. Silicone granulomatous reactions after first metatarsophalangeal hemiarthroplasty. J Bone Joint Surg [Br] 1993;75(4):637–9.
[19] Hoffman P. An operation for severe grades of contracted or clawed toes. Am J Orthop Surg 1912;9:441–9.
[20] Thomas S, Kinninmonth AW, Kumar CS. Long-term results of the modified Hoffman procedure in the rheumatoid forefoot. Surgical technique. J Bone Joint Surg [Am] 2006;88(Suppl 1): 149–57.
[21] Stockley I, Betts RP, Getty CJ, et al. A prospective study of forefoot arthroplasty. Clin Orthop 1989;248:213–8.
[22] Patsalis T, Georgousis H, Göpfert S. Long-term results of forefoot arthroplasty in patients with rheumatoid arthritis. Orthopedics 1996;19:439–47.
[23] van der Heijden KW, Rasker JJ, Jacobs JW, et al. Kates forefoot arthroplasty in rheumatoid arthritis. A 5-year follow-up study. J Rheumatol 1992;19:1545–50.
[24] Fuhrmann RA, Anders JO. The long-term results of resection arthroplasties of the first metatarsophalangeal joint in rheumatoid arthritis. Int Orthop 2001;25(5):312–6.
[25] McGarvey SR, Johnson KA. Keller arthroplasty in combination with resection arthroplasty of the lesser metatarsophalangeal joints in rheumatoid arthritis. Foot Ankle 1988;9:75–80.
[26] Vahvanen V, Piirainen H, Kettunen P. Resection arthroplasty of the metatarsophalangeal joints in rheumatoid arthritis. A follow-up study of 100 patients. Scand J Rheumatol 1980;9:257–65.
[27] Goldie I, Bremell T, Althoff B, et al. Metatarsal head resection in the treatment of the rheumatoid forefoot. Scand J Rheumatol 1983;12:106–12.
[28] Watson MS. A long-term follow-up of forefoot arthroplasty. J Bone Joint Surg [Br] 1974; 56(3):527–33.
[29] Hasselo LG, Willkens RF, Toomey HE, et al. Forefoot surgery in rheumatoid arthritis: subjective assessment of outcome. Foot Ankle 1987;8:148–51.
[30] Moynihan FJ. Arthrodesis of the metatarsophalangeal joint of the great toe. J Bone Joint Surg [Br] 1967;49(3):544–51.
[31] Neufeld SK, Parks BG, Naseef GS, et al. Arthrodesis of the first metatarsophalangeal joint: a biomechanical study comparing memory compression staples, cannulated screws, and a dorsal plate. Foot Ankle Int 2002;23(2):97–101.
[32] Huges J, Grace D, Clark P, et al. Metatarsal head excision for rheumatoid arthritis. 4 year follow-up of 68 feet with and without hallux fusion. Acta Orthop Scand 1991;62(1):63–6.
[33] Grondal L, Brostrom E, Wretenberg P, et al. Arthrodesis versus Mayo resection: the management of the first metatarsophalangeal joint in reconstruction of the rheumatoid forefoot. J Bone Joint Surg [Br] 2006;88(7):914–9.
[34] Mulcahy D, Daniels TR, Lau JT, et al. Rheumatoid forefoot deformity: a comparison study of 2 functional methods of reconstruction. J Rheumatol 2003;30(7):1440–50.
[35] Beauchamp CG, Kirby T, Rudge SR, et al. Fusion of the first metatarsophalangeal joint in forefoot arthroplasty. Clin Orthop 1984;190:249–53.
[36] Vandeputte G, Steenwerckx A, Mulier T, et al. Dereymaeker G forefoot reconstruction in rheumatoid arthritis patients: Keller-Lelievre-Hoffmann versus arthrodesis MTP1-Hoffmann. Foot Ankle Int 1999;20(7):438–43.
[37] Swanson AB, Lunmden RM, Swanson G de G. Silicone implant arthroplasty of the great toe: a review of single stem and flexible hinge implants. Clin Orthop Relat Res 1979;142: 30–43.
[38] Swanson AB. Implant arthroplasty for the great toe joint. Clin Orthop Relat Res 1972;85: 75–81.

[39] Beckenbaugh RD, Dobyns JH, Llnscbeld RL, et al. Review and analysis of silicone-rubber metacarpophalangeal implants. J Bone Joint Surg [Am] 1976;58:483–7.

[40] Aptekar RG, Davie JM. Cattail HS. Foreign body reaction to silicone rubber: complication of a finger joint implant. Clin Orthop 1974;98:231–2.

[41] Sethu A, D'Netto DC, Ramakrishna B. Swanson's silastic implants in great toes. J Bone Joint Surg [Br] 1980;62:83–5.

[42] Gordon M, Bullough PG. Synovial and osseous inflammation in failed silicone-rubber prostheses: a report of six cases. J Bone Joint Surg [Am] 1982;64:574–80.

[43] Evans G, Burke FD, Bartoui NJA. Comparison of conservative treatment and silicone replacement arthroplasty in Kienbock's disease. J Hand Surg [Br] 1986;ll:98–102.

[44] Christie AJ, Weinberger KA, Dietrich M. Silicone lymph-adenopathy and synovitis; complications of silicone elastomer finger joint prosthesis. JAMA 1977;237:1463–544.

[45] Kircher T. Silicone lymphadenopathy: a complication of silicone elastomer finger joint prosthesis. Hum Pathol 1980;11:240–4.

[46] Weinstock RE, Bass SJ, Wolfson AF, et al. Osseous engulfment of a silicone prosthesis with foreign body reaction. J Am Podiatry Assoc 1984;74:80–8.

[47] Verhaar J, Bulstra S, Walenkamp G. Silicone arthroplasty for hallux rigidus, implant wear and osteolysis. Acta Orthop Scand 1989;60:30–3.

[48] Verhaar J, Vermeulen A, Bulstra St, et al. Bone reaction to silicone metatarsophalangeal joint-1 hemiprosthesis. Clin Orthop Rel Res 1989;245:228–32.

[49] Wanivenhaus A, Lintner F, Wurnig C, et al. Long term reaction of the osseous bed around silicone implants. Arch Orthop Trauma Surg 1991;110:146–50.

[50] Yamashina M, Moatamad F. Peri-articular reactions to microscopic erosion of silicone-polymer implants. Am J Surg Pathol 1985;9:215–9.

[51] Sollitto RJ, Shonkweiler W. Silicone shard formations: a product of implant arthroplasty. J Foot Surg 1984;23:362–5.

[52] McCarthy DJ, Kershisinik W, O'Donnell E. The histopathology of silicone elastomer implant failure in podiatric surgery. J Am Podiatr Med Assoc 1986;76:247–65.

[53] Jasim KA, Wecrasinghe BD. Silicone lymphadenopathy, synovitis and osteitis complicating big toe SILASTIC® prostheses. J R Coll Surg Edinb 1987;32:29–33.

[54] Sheil WC, Jason M. Granulomatous inguinal lymphadenopathy after bilateral metatarsophalangeal joint silicone arthroplasty. Foot Ankle 1986;6:216–8.

[55] Lim WT, Landrum K, Weinberger B. Silicone lymphadenitis secondary to implant degeneration. J Foot Surg 1983;22:243–6.

[56] Groff GD, Schmed AR, Taylor TH. Silicone-induced adenopathy eight years after metacarpophalangeal arthroplasty. Arthritis Rheum 1981;24:1578–81.

[57] NaIbandlan RM, Swansea AR, Maupla BK. Long-term silicone implant arthroplasty. JAMA 1983;50:1195–8.

[58] Moeckle BH, Sculco TP, Alexiades MM, et al. The double-stemmed silicone-rubber implant for rheumatoid arthritis of the first metatarsophalangeal joint. Long-term results. J Bone Joint Surg [Am] 1992;74(4):564–70.

[59] Sebold EJ, Cracchiolo A 3rd. Use of titanium grommets in silicone implant arthroplasty of the hallux metatarsophalangeal joint. Foot Ankle Int 1996;17(3):145–51.

[60] Swanson AB, de Groot Swanson G, Ishikawa H. Use of grommets for flexible implant resection arthroplasty of the metacarpophalangeal joint. Clin Orthop Relat Res 1997;342:22–33.

[61] Shankar NS, Asaad SS, Craxford A. Hinged silastic implants of the great toe. Clin Orthop Relat Res 1991;272:227–34.

[62] Kampner SL. Long term experience with total joint prosthetic replacement for the arthritic great toe. Bull Hosp Jt Dis Orthop Inst 1987;47:153–75.

[63] Granberry WM, Noble PC, Bishop JO, et al. Use of a hinged silicone prosthesis for replacement arthroplasty of the first metatarsophalangeal joint. J Bone Joint Surg Am 1991;73(10):1453–9.

[64] Holt G, Miller N, Kelly MP, et al. Retention of the patella in total knee arthroplasty for rheumatoid arthritis. Joint Bone Spine 2006;73(5):523–6.

ELSEVIER
SAUNDERS

Foot Ankle Clin N Am
12 (2007) 417–433

FOOT AND
ANKLE CLINICS

Surgery of the Lesser Toes in Rheumatoid Arthritis: Metatarsal Head Resection

Andrew P. Molloy, MBChB, FRCS(Tr&Orth)*,
Mark S. Myerson, MD

*The Institute for Foot and Ankle Reconstructive Surgery, Mercy Medical Centre,
301 St. Paul Place, Baltimore, MD 21202, USA*

Rheumatoid arthritis is a systemic autoimmune inflammatory disease that has a prevalence of 0.5% to 1% in North America and Europe [1]. This chronic and progressive disease is polyarticular, usually with a symmetric distribution. The American Rheumatism Association has defined diagnostic criteria for its diagnosis, with four out of seven symptoms needing to be present to confirm the diagnosis. The first four categories need to have been present for at least 6 weeks: morning stiffness, arthritis in at least three joint areas associated with swelling (soft-tissue swelling or effusion, not bony overgrowth alone), symmetric arthritis, rheumatoid nodules, and serum rheumatoid factor positive [2].

Sixteen percent to 19% of patients treated for rheumatoid arthritis have symptoms in their feet and ankles as their presenting complaint [3,4]. The overall prevalence of symptoms in the foot and ankle has been reported as between 85% and 94% [3].

Forefoot arthroplasty by resection of the metatarsal heads was first described by Hoffman [5] in 1912. He described the technique of metatarsal head resection through a single plantar curved incision. Since then there have been many modifications described, including differing incisions, dermoplasty, additional bone resection from the phalanges, how much of the metatarsal head should be resected, arthroplasty with sparing of the metatarsal head and resection of the phalanges alone, how the extensors tendons are treated, and whether fixation is necessary.

---

* Corresponding author. 7 Croome Drive, West Kirby, Wirral, CH48 8AD, England, UK.

E-mail address: orthoblue@aol.com (A.P. Molloy).

1083-7515/07/$ - see front matter © 2007 Elsevier Inc. All rights reserved.
doi:10.1016/j.fcl.2007.05.001 *foot.theclinics.com*

This article focuses on the pathoanatomic basis of the deformities, a review of techniques and results in the published literature, the 'authors' preferred technique, and potential complications of forefoot arthroplasty surgery.

Pathologic and anatomic basis of lesser toe deformity

The typical deformities encountered in the rheumatoid forefoot are joint and soft-tissue swelling, hallux valgus, and dorsal subluxation or dislocation of the proximal phalanges on the metatarsal heads with or without fixed claw toe deformity. These forefoot deformities can often be associated with dorsal, medial, or lateral deviation of the toes; in fact, almost any conceivable deformity may occur in the toes. Clawing of the toes is usually present, and although initially flexible, these become progressively fixed in flexion at the proximal interphalangeal joint. These deformities are associated with plantar displacement of the metatarsal heads, distal displacement of the plantar fat pad, thick painful callosities, and possible ulceration under the prominent metatarsal heads. There may be additional fat pad atrophy either caused by the disease process itself or as a secondary effect from pharmacologic treatment.

The pathologic basis of rheumatoid arthritis is secondary to pannus formation. This chronic and invasive synovitis causes deformities by way of two mechanisms. First is through the release of degradative enzymes by way of the inflammatory cascade. The inflamed synovium is initially confined to the periarticular recesses of the joints [6]. Here it causes the typical radiologic changes of marginal erosions in early disease. As the synovium becomes more hypertrophic, hyperplastic, and inflamed by acute and chronic phases of inflammation, it spreads over the articular portion of the joints. There is then enzymatic degradation of the articular cartilage together with apparent bone loss. This appearance is worsened by the hyperemia-induced osteoporosis [7]. The articular loss is typically initially from the dorsal aspect of the metatarsal head. There is also enzymatic degradation of the normal supporting and stabilizing structures of the joint.

The second process by which the typical deformities are caused is attributable to the volume effect of the edematous, hypertrophic, and hyperplastic synovium. This causes stretching of ligaments and the capsular supportive structures. These structures lose their function, thereby affecting joint stability. The direction of joint instability depends on which area of the joint is affected, although the thin dorsal supporting structures are most at risk. If one of the collateral ligaments is affected, then obviously a crossover toe deformity ensues.

The effect of the synovitis, especially the loss of the dorsal bony and soft-tissue stabilizing structures, causes progressive dorsal subluxation of the proximal phalanges. This has various anatomic effects that contribute to the deterioration of the deformity. The primary plantar flexors of the metatarsophalangeal joints are the interossei and the lumbricals. Their mechanical axis as they insert into the base of the proximal phalanx is plantar to the rotational axis of the metatarsophalangeal joint, thereby producing a flexion moment on their contracture. On dorsal subluxation of the proximal phalanges, however, the axis of the interossei is transferred to the dorsal side of the rotational axis of the joint, causing them to become weak extensors or, at best, functionless [8]. The lumbrical tendons do not subluxate, because they are tethered under the transverse metatarsal ligament; however, they also become largely inefficient because of the magnitude of the acute angulation that occurs from where they pass under the transverse metatarsal ligament up to their insertion point (Fig. 1). Resistance to the dorsally deforming forces is reduced as active flexion of the metatarsophalangeal joint is lost.

The pathologic position of the toes causes further deformity at the interphalangeal joints because of further muscle imbalance and altered function. The extensor digitorum brevis, and in particular, extensor digitorum longus, function with greatest efficiency and strength when the phalanges are in a neutral or flexed position. Their function is therefore diminished by the relative hyperextension caused by the dorsal subluxation or dislocation. In contrast, especially with subluxation, the flexor digitorum longus and flexor digitorum brevis still function.

The plantar fat pad is attached to the plantar plate by way of fibrous septae between the plantar plate and the plantar skin. The plantar plate, which is the distal insertion of the plantar aponeurosis, has a thick cartilaginous attachment to the base of the proximal phalanx but only a thin, flimsy

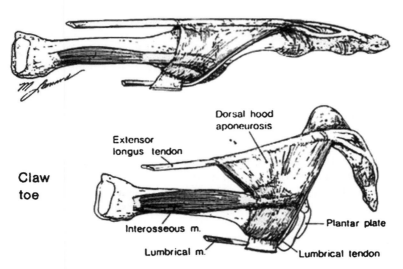

Fig. 1. Tendinous relationships to the metatarsophalangeal joint in normal and clawed toes (*Modified from* Myerson MS. Arthroplasty of the second toe [Fig. 1]. Semin Arthroplasty 1992;3(1):31–8; with permission.)

attachment to the metatarsal neck [8,9]. As the proximal phalanx dorsally subluxates, the attachment of the plantar plate to the metatarsal neck tears because of its relative weakness as compared with the attachment to the proximal phalanx. This causes the plantar plate and its attached fat pad to displace distally as they accompany the proximal phalanx to its deformed position. The fat pad therefore comes to lie anterior to the metatarsal head rather than covering its plantar aspect.

This uncovering of the metatarsal heads is accentuated by depression of the metatarsal heads [9]. This is caused by the slips of plantar fascia to each metatarsal sliding dorsally on either side of the metatarsal heads as the plantar plate moves with the proximal phalanx. As they tighten, they therefore depress the metatarsal heads by their dorsal position with respect to the rotational axis of the metatarsophalangeal joints. There is also a secondary plunger effect of the metatarsals caused by the tethering of the plantar plate by the transverse metatarsal ligaments [9].

Historical aspects of metatarsal head resection

Hoffman [5] first published his method of pan-metatarsal head resection in 1912. He described the use of a single transverse curved plantar incision behind the level of the webs of the toes. He stated that sufficient bone needed to be resected to permit free motion between the phalangeal bases and the metatarsal stumps, which inevitably meant that the entire metatarsal head and part of the neck needed to be excised. He believed that extensor tenotomies were unnecessary because of the relaxation in the soft tissues caused by the shortening of the metatarsals. No Kirschner wires nor any form of splinting were used in the postoperative period.

In 1959 Fowler [10] described the use of a dorsal transverse incision with short longitudinal extensions along the shafts of the first and fifth metatarsals. The proximal halves of the phalanges were excised along with trimming of the metatarsal heads. This trimming involved at least a plantar condylectomy, but usually a more extensive excision was required. A second incision excising an ellipse of skin from the plantar surface was used to help relocate the plantar fat pad. No extensor tenotomies or lengthening procedures were performed. A year later Clayton [11] published his technique of approaching the resection through a straighter dorsal transverse incision (although he states that he had previously used multiple incisions but found it more preferable to use a transverse incision instead). The resection involved the metatarsal heads and the proximal half of the phalangeal base, except sometimes in the case of the fifth metatarsal. The extensors were transected in severe deformities. Splintage was simply in the form of a compression dressing. Kates and colleagues [12] published their modification in 1967 in which the approach was by way of a curved plantar incision. A thorough pan-metatarsal head resection was described, together with excision of an ellipse of skin for further control of the deformity correction. Splintage was provided by a Kirschner wire for the first metatarsophalangeal joint and a plaster cast moulded into plantar flexion for the lesser toes.

The use of three dorsal longitudinal incisions was first published by Larmon [13] in 1951 but on a wider scale by Lipscomb [14] in 1968. Lipscomb's [14] technique of forefoot arthroplasty involved a Keller procedure with a partial or total proximal phalangectomy, a metatarsal head plantar condylectomy, and an extensor tenotomy for each of the lateral four toes. Maclean and Silver [15] modified Dwyer's [16] method of forefoot arthroplasty using a first metatarsophalangeal joint arthrodesis, lesser metatarsal head resection, and lesser proximal interphalangeal joint arthrodesis by describing transposition of the transected extensor tendon into the cavity of the excised first metatarsophalangeal joint to help prevent loss of position by dorsal contracture of the extensor tendons. Most modifications of forefoot arthroplasty since have concerned the varying methods of first metatarsophalangeal arthrodesis, joint replacement, and resection arthroplasty together with varying methods of their fixation.

The only other method of resection arthroplasty is the Stainsby procedure, the results of which were first published by Briggs and Stainsby [17] in 2001. This technique preserves the metatarsal heads. Four V incisions (with the apices pointing laterally) are used to approach the partial proximal phalangectomies, which are performed at the level of the phalangeal neck. The dislocated plantar plate is freed from the metatarsal head and relocated, followed by tenodesis of the tenotomized extensors to their respective flexor tendons. Fixation is achieved with intramedullary Kirschner wires.

Theoretic basis of techniques

There are several approaches that have been advocated for resection of the lesser metatarsal heads, and each of them have theoretic advantages and disadvantages (Fig. 2A–E). The original description by Hoffman [5] was of a curved plantar incision, with Fowler [10] and Kates and colleagues [11] advocating the addition of a dermoplasty. The advantages of this approach are that it allows excellent direct visualization of the metatarsal heads and it allows excision of the calluses and the dermoplasty assisting in reducing the deformity. There are certainly risks for a hypertrophic keratotic plantar scar, however, and if enough bone is not excised, the resulting excessive longitudinal traction may cause a wound dehiscence. Rates of failure of primary healing can vary from 5% to 36% [18,19]. Patients need to be nonweightbearing on the forefoot until the wound has healed, although this can be avoided by the use of a wedged heel postoperative shoe. Obviously further incisions are necessary if the extensor tendons are to be addressed. Fowler described a combined dorsal and plantar approach that combines the excellent exposure of the dorsal transverse incision and a plantar dermoplasty. Although this combined approach has potential benefits, it also has the potential risks for both. Although Fowler's [10] original article describes

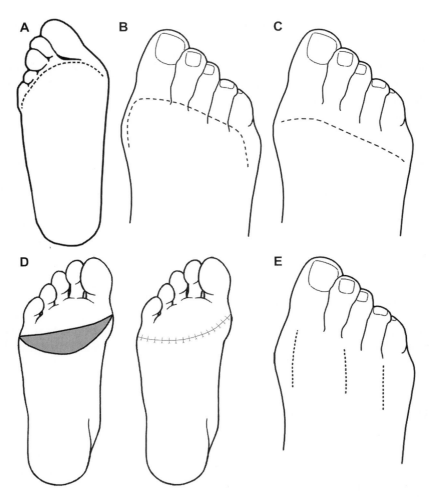

Fig. 2. Approaches to lesser metatarsal head resections. (*A*) Hoffman. (*B*) Fowler (used additional plantar dermoplasty; see [*D*]). (*C*) Clayton. (*D*) Kates et al. (*E*) Dorsal longitudinal.

a 5% incidence of wound problems, a later series by Barton [19] reported problems in 46% of patients. Clayton [11] first described the use of a sole dorsal transverse incision, which still has widespread use today. This avoids the problem of the hyperkeratotic scar but still carries the same complications of wound problems [11,19]. It still allows excellent visualization of the metatarsal heads and of the extensors. In using either of the transverse approaches one has to be certain to excise enough bone so as to not place the wound under any undue longitudinal tension and thereby attempt to avoid a wound dehiscence. The use of three dorsal longitudinal incisions has been widely popularized since its inception by Larmon [13] and then Lipscomb [14]. A lower incidence of wound complications is reported with this approach; 7% to 18% as compared with 5% to 42% from the previously described approaches [18–21]. The exposure is obviously not as wide with this approach, although its proponents argue that it is sufficient even in the most severe cases. Fowler and Clayton [10,11] argued that this more limited exposure could lead to incorrect bone resection, although this has not been borne out in more recent studies, with Coughlin [22] describing 96% accuracy in recreation of the metatarsal parabola. Great care, however, needs to be taken with obtaining adequate exposure using this approach, because over-retraction leads to wound problems. Retraction should only be on deep tissues and not on the skin. The only other caveat to this approach is potentially in the presence of preoperative vasculitis with regard to the skin bridges between the dorsal longitudinal incisions.

Many of the original investigators stated that it was unnecessary to divide or lengthen the extensor tendons and their preservation could lead to improved function. There is residual dorsiflexion of the metatarsophalangeal joint in up to 87% of cases when the extensors are left intact [18–20]. Coughlin [22], however, an advocator of leaving the extensor tendons intact, on follow-up of a mean of 74 months found a 7% redislocation rate in the sagittal plane and incidence of 16% subluxation and dislocation in the axial plane. The Stainsby procedure, which involves an extensor tenotomy and tenodesis to the flexors, has been reported as having a 26% incidence of the toes not touching the ground.

Investigators [21–23] have described using bone-cutting rongeurs or a saw to osteotomize the neck. Rongeurs can certainly cause crushing of the bone if osteopenia is only minimal, and it can therefore be more time-consuming to remove the shards. There have been no reports of differing levels of heterotrophic ossification between the two methods. The disadvantages of using a saw are that wider exposure is necessary to avoid skin or soft-tissue damage and that retraction needs to be especially thorough if a plantar approach is used so as to avoid damage to the neurovascular structures.

The original advocators of forefoot arthroplasty recommended no splintage, or at most a plaster cast, for the toes. They did, however, describe a loss of position in up to 87% of cases [18–20]. In more recent series, rates of loss of position have been as poor as 60% [24]. It should be considered standard technique to transfix the toes with Kirschner wires in view of such good long-term results as in Coughlin's [22] series. This is confirmed in a small study comparing syndactylization and Kirschner wire transfixing at more than 2 years of follow-up, which showed better cosmesis, function, and plantar pressure movements in the transfixed group (IA Alexander, personal communication, 1991).

Authors' preferred technique

The operation is performed under twilight sedation and local anesthetic blockade of the popliteal, common peroneal, and saphenous nerves using a mixture of 1% lidocaine and 0.25% Marcaine. Epinephrine is not used in conjunction with the local anesthetic for fear of vascular compromise, especially if there is a background of rheumatoid-induced vasculitis. A nerve stimulator is used for accurate placement of the popliteal and common peroneal blocks.

A tourniquet is not normally used. This is because this practice encourages gentler treatment of the soft tissues and more thoroughness in achieving hemostasis. This is of paramount importance in trying to avoid complications of wound hematoma, infection, or dehiscence. It also allows for visualization of the vascularity of the lesser toes once they have been reduced and transfixed. If there is a problem with vascularity, this can be dealt with in prompt fashion while still under sterile conditions.

The choice of approach and incisions used for lesser metatarsal head resections in the patient who has rheumatoid arthritis is determined by the magnitude of deformity and quality of soft tissues. The standard approach is to use two dorsal longitudinal incisions, one between the second and third metatarsals and one between the fourth and fifth metatarsals (Fig. 3). Generous incisions should be used to prevent excessive retraction of soft tissues while trying to get adequate exposure of the metatarsal heads and necks. If plantar ulceration is present, this dorsal approach can still be used. The metatarsal head resection would be performed in a standard fashion, followed by excision of the ulcer edges. An antibiotic impregnated swab is passed from

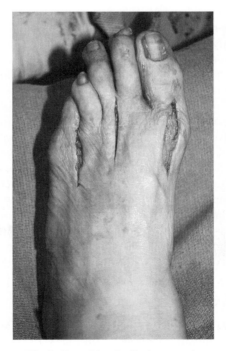

Fig. 3. Dorsal longitudinal approach.

dorsal to plantar in a repetitive fashion almost like a dental-flossing action. This plantar wound is left open and heals by secondary intention.

If there is a general paucity of the soft tissues or if there is edema present and certainly if there is any suspicion of cutaneous vascular compromise, a dorsal transverse incision is used. It is also used if there is a particularly severe deformity, because this approach provides easier exposure of the metatarsal heads in these conditions. If this approach is used, however, one must be sure that the wound is not under tension on closure, because this can promote wound-healing problems. The authors' experience, however, is that these problems are rare if sufficient bone is resected to provide a tension-free reduction. A plantar approach, including excision of an ellipse of plantar skin, is rarely used (Fig. 4A,B). The only real indication is if it is a particularly severe and fixed deformity. This presentation is rare in patients who have rheumatoid arthritis and is normally associated with seronegative arthropathies or in neuropathies (such as in spina bifida) and secondary to diabetes mellitus. If this approach is used dorsal percutaneous extensor tenotomies should be used.

The lesser metatarsal head resections are performed first, followed by the first metatarsophalangeal joint arthrodesis. This is because it is easier to determine the appropriate length of the hallux and therefore the amount of bone resection necessary once the lesser toes have been addressed. It also avoids compromise of the stability of the fusion by inadvertent manipulation of the hallux.

The dorsal approach to the lesser metatarsal heads is performed through the aforementioned two incisions that extend from the cleft of the respective web space for at least 4 cm. Retraction of the skin and soft tissues is only

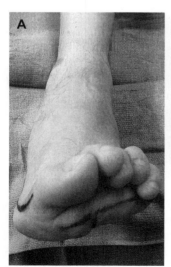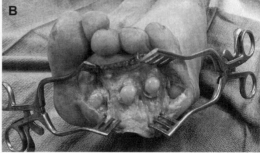

Fig. 4. Plantar approach. (*A*) Skin marking for incisions. (*B*) Metatarsal heads exposed.

performed in one incision at a time and preferably only on one side of the incision at a time. Army and Navy/Langebach retractors are used rather than self-retaining retractors. These measures prevent over-retraction and trauma to the soft tissues. The approach is deepened down to each extensor tendon, which is divided under tension at the proximal end of the wound. They are each clamped with a hemostat and dissected distally to the base of the proximal phalanges. They can then be pulled through the web space medial to their respective metatarsal. The hemostat is left to hang free on the plantar surface of the foot, working as an excellent retractor, facilitating exposure of the metatarsophalangeal joints.

A capsulotomy of the metatarsophalangeal joint is performed together with dissection to free the base of the proximal phalanx, including cutting the collateral ligaments. The joint is not always easy to visualize if there is a frank dislocation, but it must be reduced before the osteotomy is performed. Once the base of the proximal phalanx has been freed, a curved periosteal elevator is introduced into the metatarsophalangeal joint. Plantar-directed pressure together with longitudinal traction introduces the head into the incision. Occasionally this maneuver crushes the metatarsal head because of the rheumatoid-induced osteopenia. This is not problematic providing all free fragments are meticulously removed. The curved periosteal elevator is then used to free around the plantar surface to facilitate its removal in its entirety. The elevator is left in this position, because it helps gain control of the metatarsal head during the neck cut.

An oscillating saw is used to cut the neck at the flare of the metaphyseal–diaphyseal junction. The direction of this cut is plantar oblique from the dorsal surface. Care must be taken over the excursion of the saw blade and especially not to skirt off the metatarsal, as this greatly traumatizes the soft tissues. The head is grasped with a towel clip, rotated, and removed in its entirety (Fig. 5). Occasionally some remaining soft tissues, including the plantar plate, prevent this removal and should be freed using sharp dissection.

Persistent deformity at the interphalangeal joints following resection of the metatarsal heads is addressed by three different methods. If this is a flexible deformity, closed osteoclasis is preferred. If the deformity is fixed at all, a joint resection arthroplasty is performed, normally through a dorsal longitudinal incision. This is preferred to arthrodesis, because it helps preserve length of the toes with equal results. An interphalangeal joint arthrodesis, by the same approach, is usually reserved for revision surgery. A Kirschner wire is used for fixation in whichever method is used.

A plantar extensor tenodesis is performed to help prevent dorsal contracture and thereby loss of position. A Kirschner wire is passed antegrade from the base of the proximal phalanx. This obviously also holds the position of the interphalangeal joints. Occasionally if there is a mild residual deformity the wire may not pass through the tip of the toe, but this does not cause any problems. A hemostat is used to pass the tendon underneath the

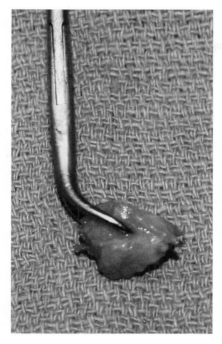

Fig. 5. Metatarsal head removed in its entirety.

metatarsal neck. The Kirschner wire is then passed retrograde, through the extensor tendon, and down the medullary canal of the metatarsal. Because of the relative osteopenia, stability of the Kirschner wires can only be achieved by driving the wires into the cuneiforms or the cuboid. Because of the curved nature of the fifth metatarsal the wire sometimes passes out through the lateral cortex of the metatarsal shaft, and this provides adequate purchase. The authors have had no incidences of snapped wires with this technique and have found less incidence of wire loosening. Rarely passage of the wires together with correction of the deformity can cause vasospasm. If this is slow to resolve, nitroglycerine paste can be applied. If this still does not resolve on the table, the wire must be removed. An exacerbating factor for vasospasm can be if the toes are transfixed in too dorsiflexed a position, which kinks the vessel. By placing the toes into a slightly plantarflexed position it may still be possible to transfix the toes. If it is done in this position the Kirschner wires exit through the dorsal surface (Fig. 6). If no positional change is necessary or it is of no avail, the position is held by tape strapping or a splint made from petroleum gauze, which gradually hardens with exposure to air.

If the disease process affects the first metatarsophalangeal joint, arthrodesis is performed in conjunction with the lesser metatarsal head resection. The authors' standard approach for this procedure is by way of a direct

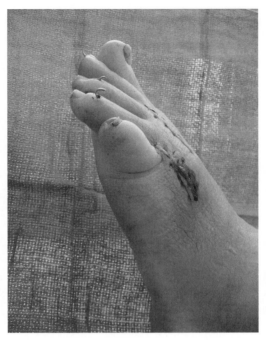

Fig. 6. Flexed position of toes with dorsally exiting wires caused by vasospasm secondary to severe deformity correction.

medial approach. This allows a sufficiently large skin bridge between this incision and the one placed between the second and third metatarsals. The bone resection for the first metatarsophalangeal joint arthrodesis is performed by using a 5-mm oval high-speed burr to fashion reciprocating cup and cone shapes. The standard technique for fixation of the arthrodesis is two crossed 4.5-mm cannulated screws. If there is severe osteopenia or bone defects present that would make this method of fixation difficult, a single 4.5-mm cannulated screw is used together with a neutralization plate. The authors have recently noted that a locking plate (Hand Innovations System, Depuy, Warsaw, IN) provides excellent fixation and there have been no instances of nonunion using this system. In the presence of extremely poor quality bone in which arthrodesis is necessary, two Steinman pins may be used. It is usually necessary to leave these in place for 8 to 10 weeks. If the first metatarsophalangeal joint is unaffected, surgery on it is unnecessary. If conservative management of this joint is followed, however, the position of the hallux needs to be closely monitored. If it starts to drift into valgus, then it abuts the second toe, causing a recurrence of deformity that can be challenging to treat. If the first metatarsophalangeal joint is spared, closer consideration does need to be given as to whether it would be more appropriate to carry out joint-sparing surgery on the lesser toes, such as Weil or Maceira osteotomies. The choice of approach for these surgeries would be by way of three dorsal longitudinal or a single dorsal transverse incision. The former is the more likely to be used, because the minimal shortening can be a cause of undue tension on the wound with the aforementioned ensuing complications. Generally the authors are not proponents of resection arthroplasty of the first metatarsophalangeal joint for rheumatoid disease. Although some investigators have shown equivocal results between resection arthroplasty at the early to mid-term stage, there have been an equal number of investigators who have found a rapid recurrence of deformity. From the authors' experience with revision arthroplasty for the rheumatoid forefoot, most patients have had a resection arthroplasty (in addition to having had the extensor tendons intact) with the recurrence occurring a large proportion of the time after 5 years.

Revision forefoot arthroplasty is a challenging procedure. There is usually cutaneous thinning and an element of subcutaneous fibrosis. Great care needs to be taken over obtaining exposure and prevention of over-retraction. The approach used in the index operation need not influence the approach used for the revision surgery, providing the index operation was more than approximately 2 years ago. The normal parabola of metatarsal length needs to be diligently recreated. One should err on the side of larger bony resection from the metatarsals so as to prevent further recurrence. Although this obviously shortens the toe, patients would prefer to have a shorter toe rather than a deforming one. A first metatarsophalangeal arthrodesis is inevitably performed. If revising a previous arthrodesis, the osteotomy is performed with a crescentic oscillating saw (Fig. 7). The plane of the cut can be altered to help with correction of deformity. If a resection arthroplasty or prosthetic arthroplasty has previously been performed, the

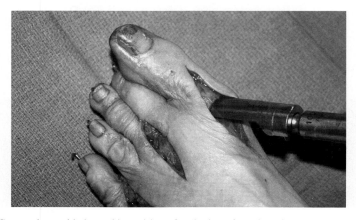

Fig. 7. Crescentic saw blade used in revision of malunion of previous first metatarsophalangeal arthrodesis.

bone defect, which can be huge, needs to be filled with cancellous graft and possibly supplemented by other osteoconductive and osteoinductive materials.

The surgical incisions are normally closed with nylon sutures, because the paucity of the soft tissues rarely holds a subcutaneous absorbable suture. The wounds are dressed in standard fashion with a simple wool and crepe compression dressing. The patients are allowed to bear weight as tolerated in a postoperative shoe with an elevated wedge heel, although they are encouraged to keep the affected limb elevated as much as possible. Sutures are removed at 2 weeks, with the Kirschner wires being kept in place for 6 weeks, when they are removed in the office (Figs. 8 and 9).

Results and complications

There are many ways of describing results of lesser metatarsal head resection in the literature, with success being described by subjective, objective, functional, and radiographic methods. The most robust study seems to be Coughlin's [22] long-term study, which used the American Orthopedic Foot and Ankle Society (AOFAS) scoring system [25] for assessment at a mean of 74 months postsurgery, although this method was obviously not open to investigators before its inception in 1994. Overall satisfaction

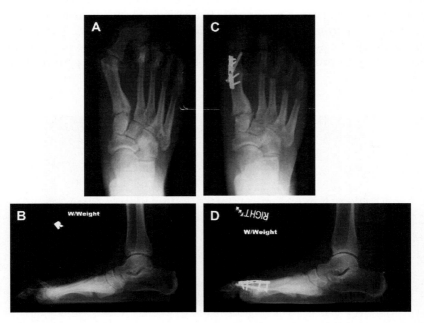

Fig. 8. Radiographs of marked deformity in a 64-year-old man. (*A*) Preoperative AP. (*B*) Preoperative lateral. (*C*) 6 weeks postoperative AP. (*D*) 6 weeks postoperative lateral.

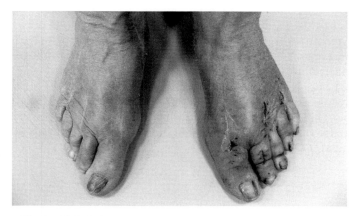

Fig. 9. Clinical photograph at 6 weeks post surgery for the left foot.

levels vary from 72% to 100% at between 18 and 74 months [10,12,15,19,20,22,26]. There is one outlying study from this group in which first metatarsophalangeal arthrodesis was performed. Hulse and Thomas [27] found that less than 60% of patients were satisfied at 6.6 years. In studies in which resection arthroplasty was performed, satisfaction levels ranged from 32% to 67% [20,28–30]. Where mentioned separately, function was found to have improved in 91% to 97% of patients [12,18,21]. Mann and Schakel [21] reported that 60% of women were able to wear high heels of 1.5 in and 50% of men could wear dress shoes, whereas Bitzan and colleagues [31] reported that 93% of patients were able to wear normal shoes after forefoot arthroplasty.

Complications can include infection, wound dehiscence, hematoma, metatarsalgia, plantar callosities, loss of position, and amputation, although fortunately the latter is extremely rare. The complication rates differ based on which approach is used, as dealt with in the section on the theoretic basis of techniques. There does historically seem to be fewer complications if dorsal longitudinal incisions are used and Kirschner wire fixation is used. The rate of reoperation varies from 5% to 40%, and again, this rate seems to be higher if resection arthroplasty is performed on the first metatarsophalangeal joint [20,22,26,27]. Thordarson and colleagues [32] found that there was a failure rate of 85% if hallux metatarsophalangeal joint preservation surgery was performed. There is little published literature on how the effects of pharmacologic agents affect the complication rates. Bibbo and colleagues [33] found no statistical link between pharmacologic agents and complications in a retrospective review of 104 patients who underwent 725 procedures. In a further study Bibbo and Goldberg [33,34] found no link between infectious and healing complications and tumor necrosis factor alpha therapy.

Summary

The typical deformities in a rheumatoid forefoot of hallux valgus, depressed metatarsal heads, and dorsally subluxed or dislocated toes, cause pain because of areas of increased plantar pressure, instability, and ongoing synovitis. Lesser metatarsal head resection allows reduction of this increased pressure while providing a stable forefoot with a low rate of recurrence of deformity. This is a reproducible form of forefoot arthroplasty that has good success rates with an acceptable level of complications over long-term follow-up.

References

[1] Felson DT. Epidemiology of the rheumatic diseases. In: Koppman WJ, editor. Arthritis and allied conditions; a textbook of rheumatology. 13th edition. Baltimore (MD): Williams & Wilkins; 1997. p. 6.

[2] Arnett FC, Edworthy SM, Bloch DA, et al. The American Rheumatism Association 1987 revised criteria for the classification of rheumatoid arthritis. Arthritis Rheum 1988;31: 315–24.

[3] Vainio K. Rheumatoid foot. Clinical study with pathological and roentgenological comments. Ann Chir Gynaecol Fenn Suppl 1956;45(Suppl):1–107.

[4] Fleming A, Crown JM, Corbett M. Early rheumatoid disease. I. Onset. Ann Rheum Dis 1976;35:357–60.

[5] Hoffman MD. An operation for severe grades of contracted or clawed toes. Am J Orthop Surg 1912;9:441–9.

[6] Gold RH, Basset IW. Radiologic evaluation of the arthritic foot. Foot Ankle 1982;2:332–41.

[7] Guerra J, Resnick D. Arthritides affecting the foot: radiographic pathological correlation. Foot Ankle 1982;2:325–31.

[8] Myerson MS. Arthroplasty of the second toe. Semin Arthroplasty 1992;3(1):31–8.

[9] Stainsby GD. Pathological anatomy and dynamic effect of the displaced plantar plate and the importance of the plantar plate–deep transverse metatarsal ligament tie-bar. Ann R Coll Surg Engl 1997;79:58–68.

[10] Fowler AW. A method of forefoot reconstruction. J Bone Joint Surg Br 1959;41:507–13.

[11] Clayton ML. Surgery of the forefoot in rheumatoid arthritis. Clin Orthop 1960;16:136–40.

[12] Kates A, Kessel L, Kay A. Arthroplasty of the forefoot. J Bone Joint Surg Br 1967;49:552–7.

[13] Larmon WA. Surgical treatment of deformities of rheumatoid arthritis of the forefoot and toes. Q Bull Northwest Univ Med Sch 1951;25:39.

[14] Lipscomb PR. Surgery for rheumatoid arthritis—timing and techniques: summary. J Bone Joint Surg Am 1968;50(3):614–7.

[15] MacClean CR, Silver WA. Dwyers' operation for the rheumatoid forefoot. Foot Ankle 1981;1(6):343–7.

[16] Dwyer AE. Correction of severe toe deformities. J Bone Joint Surg Br 1970;52:192.

[17] Briggs PJ, Stainsby GD. Metatarsal head preservation in forefoot arthroplasty and the correction of severe claw toe deformity. Foot Ankle 2001;7:93–101.

[18] Stockley I, Betts RP, Getty CJM, et al. A prospective study of forefoot arthroplasty. Clin Orthop Relat Res 1989 Nov;(248):213–8.

[19] Barton NJ. Arthroplasty of the forefoot in rheumatoid arthritis. J Bone Joint Surg Br 1973; 55(1):126–33.

[20] Watson MS. A long–-term follow-up of forefoot arthroplasty. J Bone Joint Surg Br 1974;56: 527–33.

[21] Mann RA, Schakel ME II. Surgical correction of rheumatoid forefoot deformities. Foot Ankle Int 1995;16(1):1–6.

[22] Coughlin MJ. Rheumatoid forefoot reconstruction. A long-term follow-up study. J Bone Joint Surg Am 2000;82:322–41.

[23] Myerson MS. The rheumatoid foot and ankle. In: Myerson MS, editor. Reconstructive foot and ankle surgery. Baltimore (MD): Elsevier Saunders; 2005. p. 475–86.

[24] Saltrick KR, Alter SA, Catanzariti A. Pan metatarsal head resection: retrospective analysis and literature review. J Foot Surg 1989;28(4):340–5.

[25] Kitaoka HB, Alexander IJ, Adelaar RS, et al. Clinical rating systems for the ankle–hindfoot, midfoot, hallux, and lesser toes. Foot Ankle Int 1994;15:349–53.

[26] Hamalainen M, Raunio P. Long-term followup of rheumatoid forefoot surgery. Clin Orthop Relat Res 1997;340:34–8.

[27] Hulse N, Thomas AMC. Metatarsal head resection in the rheumatoid foot: 5-year follow-up with and without resection of the first metatarsal head. J Foot Ankle Surg 2006;45(2):107–12.

[28] Van der Heijden KW, Rasker JJ, Jacobs JW, et al. Kates forefoot arthroplasty in rheumatoid arthritis. A 5-year followup study. J Rheumatol 1992;19:1545–50.

[29] Vahvanen V, Piirainen H, Kettunen P. Resection arthroplasty of the metatarsophalangeal joints in rheumatoid arthritis. A follow-up study of 100 patients. Scand J Rheumatol 1980;9: 257–65.

[30] Goldie I, Bremell T, Althoff B, et al. Metatarsal head resection in the treatment of the rheumatoid forefoot. Scand J Rheumatol 1983;12:106–12.

[31] Bitzan P, Giurea A, Wanivenhaus A. Plantar pressure distribution after resection of the metatarsal heads in rheumatoid arthritis. Foot Ankle Int 1997;18(7):391–7.

[32] Thordarson DB, Aval S, Krieger L. Failure of hallux preservation surgery for rheumatoid arthritis. Foot Ankle Int 2002;23(6):486–90.

[33] Bibbo C, Andreson RA, Hodges Davies W, et al. Rheumatoid nodules and postoperative complications. Foot Ankle Int 2003;24(1):40–4.

[34] Bibbo C, Goldberg JW. Infectious and healing complications after elective orthopaedic foot and ankle surgery during tumor necrosis factor-alpha inhibition therapy. Foot Ankle Int 2005;25(5):332–5.

ELSEVIER
SAUNDERS

Foot Ankle Clin N Am
12 (2007) 435–454

FOOT AND
ANKLE CLINICS

Joint-Preserving Surgery in Rheumatoid Forefoot: Preliminary Study with More-Than-Two–Year Follow-Up

Louis Samuel Barouk, MD[a],*, Pierre Barouk, MD[b]

[a]*Polyclinique de Bourdeaux, 151 Rue du Tondu, 33000 Bordeaux, France*
[b]*Clinique St. Antoine de Padoue, 28 Rue Walter Poupot, 33000 Bordeaux, France*

As an alternative to the "classic" surgical approach to the rheumatoid forefoot, which combines a first metatarsophalangeal (MTP) fusion and lesser metatarsal head resections, the authors propose a joint-preserving surgery for rheumatoid forefoot deformities.

In most cases, by the time the rheumatoid patient visits the orthopedic clinic, the inflammatory phase of the patient's arthritis has subsided. The result is a patient who is in remission but is left with a severely impaired forefoot involving the MTP joints and metatarsal heads. The associated deformity is often severe. These disorders may be treated by applying the same principles of joint-preserving surgery that the authors use in correcting other severe static disorders of the forefoot, namely the large and harmonized shortening of all of the metatarsals [1,2]. (Such global and large shortening osteotomies were also reported by Maceira Ref. [3]). However, in some patients, the acute inflammatory phase of the arthritis persists at the time of surgical consultation, in which case the role of joint-preserving surgery must be further assessed.

Hanyu and colleagues [4] reported on a series of 75 cases of rheumatoid forefeet treated by Weil osteotomies of the lateral rays and either a MTP implant or a Mitchell osteotomy of the first ray. Rippstein [5] fused the first MTP joint routinely and performed lateral metatarsal shortening with Weil osteotomies. However, to preserve MTP joint motion, Rippstein has more recently used an extra-articular Scarf first-metatarsal osteotomy procedure, except for in the presence of severe impairment. Recently, Berg and colleagues [6] reported a review of 20 cases of joint-preserving surgery in

---

* Corresponding author.
E-mail address: samuel.barouk@wanadoo.fr (L.S. Barouk).

1083-7515/07/$ - see front matter © 2007 Elsevier Inc. All rights reserved.
doi:10.1016/j.fcl.2007.05.006

rheumatoid forefeet using Scarf and Weil osteotomies, but these were in mild cases without severe impairment of the MTP joints. The authors have been using a first-metatarsal Scarf osteotomy and Weil osteotomies of the lesser metatarsals to manage the rheumatoid forefoot since 1993 [7,8]. The goal was to bring greater accuracy to the amount, location, and technique of these metatarsal-shortening osteotomies, as well as to show that the indications for this procedure may be extended to even severely deformed joints. The current follow-up is now sufficient to assess these results and to determine the role of such joint-preserving surgery in the rheumatoid forefoot (Fig. 1).

Materials and methods

Between 1994 and 2005, the authors performed surgical corrections of rheumatoid forefoot deformity in 60 feet among 34 patients. The average follow-up was 6 years and 3 months (range: 2–12 years). There were 31 women and 3 men in the study group. The average patient age was 53.3 years. Out of the 60 feet, 55 had a Scarf osteotomy performed on the first metatarsal (92%), while 5 underwent first MTP joint fusion (8%). On the lateral rays, 240 lateral metatarsal Weil osteotomies were performed (86%) versus 34 metatarsal head resections (14%). Additional procedures are indicated below.

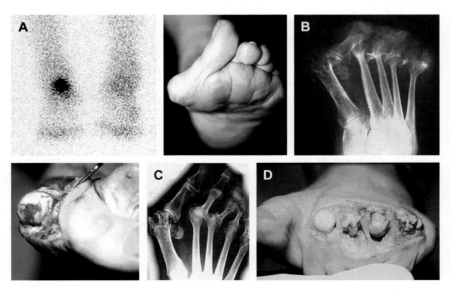

Fig. 1. The status of the rheumatoid forefoot prior to surgery. (*A, B*) The inflammatory period is finished in most cases, but the forefoot deformities are severe. (*C, D*) The MTP joints are dislocated. The metatarsal heads are also severely impaired, with cystic changes evident.

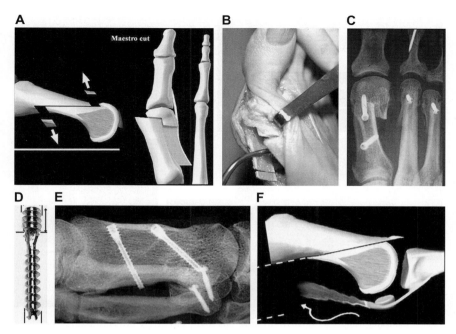

Fig. 2. Joint-preserving shortening of the first ray. (*A–C*) Scarf osteotomy, which combines shortening and a lateral shift. Note the distal cut (Maestro), which protects the lateral ligament and increases the fragment contact. The lateral shift should be mild to moderate, but the metatarsal shortening must be large. (*D–E*) The FRS screw, a modification of the Barouk screw, is particularly effective in rheumatoid forefoot bone. (*F*) Another joint-preserving procedure to shorten the 1st metatarsal (Weil osteotomy).

A complete study, including more detailed analysis and American Orthopaedic Foot & Ankle Society (AOFAS) scoring is in progress. The preliminary findings presented here establish the basis and principle of this procedure and are sufficient.to assess the results of such joint-preserving surgery.

Surgical technique: principles and practical points

The main principle is joint preservation by shortening osteotomies of all the metatarsals performed at the primary location of the rheumatoid forefoot lesions, namely the MTP joints and metatarsal heads. A Scarf osteotomy is normally performed on the first ray. A Weil osteotomy is performed on the lesser metatarsals.

For the Scarf osteotomy on the first ray (Fig. 2), the primary correction is above all shortening, combined with a moderate lateral shift and other displacements as required [9–14]. The Scarf is fixed with either Barouk or Fusion and Reconstruction System (FRS) screws (Depuy). Less often, the

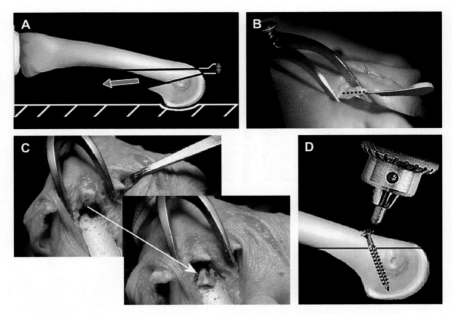

Fig. 3. Weil osteotomy. Double-layer osteotomy and fixation. (*A, B*) This double-layer bone cut is always required, above all in cases in which the shortening is very large. (*C*) In many cases, we have to cut the metatarsal perpendicularly to the shaft; note the removed slice of bone. (*D*) Fixation with a twist-off screw (Depuy), or a 2.5 FR screw (Depuy).

authors use the Weil first-metatarsal distal shortening osteotomy to correct the first ray deformity [15,16].

On the lesser metatarsals, the Weil osteotomy (Figs. 3–4) [17–19] is modified by the addition of a second saw cut with removal of a thin trapezoidal section of bone to avoid plantar translation of the metatarsal head. Fixation is by either a Twist-Off Screw or by the 2.5 FRS screw.

This metatarsal shortening must have the following features:

- It has to be large. The average shortening on the first ray in this series was 11 mm (range:7–15 mm). The average shortening on the lateral rays was 13 mm (range: 8–17 mm) (Fig. 4).

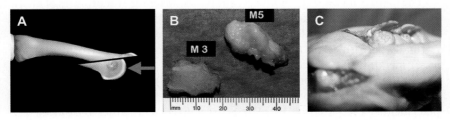

Fig. 4. Weil osteotomy. The proximal translation must be large. Average shortening is 15 mm.

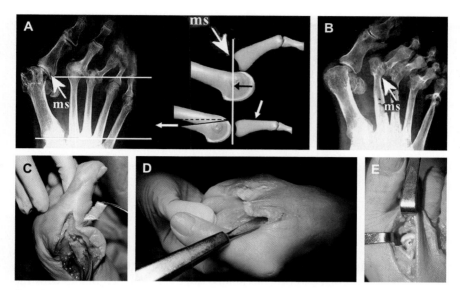

Fig. 5. Assessment of metatarsal shortening: the MS point. (*A*, *B*) Preoperative assessment. The MS point is located at the proximal part of the proximal phalanx of the most impaired ray. (*C–E*) Intraoperative adjustment. On the first ray, 60° of dorsiflexion is achieved at the 1st MTP joint. On the lateral rays, the spatula releases the attachments of the plantar plate to the metatarsal neck so that the head can be translated as far as necessary for the MTP dislocation to be corrected without any tightness.

- It must be focused on the metatarsal shortening point (MS point) (Fig. 5) [20]. This point is assessed preoperatively on the antero-posterior radiographs or, if required, on the oblique view. The MS point is determined by first analyzing the most impaired or deformed ray of the foot. The MS point is the projection of the most proximal part of the base of the proximal phalanx on to its corresponding metatarsal. The amount of metatarsal shortening required to reduce the deformity is the distance between this point and the distal end of the metatarsal head; the other metatarsals are then adjusted around this ray as described below. This preoperative assessment usually shows that all of the metatarsals require shortening (Figs. 6A–E).
- While shortening all five metatarsals, the metatarsal curve must be respected following the rules of Tanaka and colleagues [21], Maestro and colleagues [22]. The first and second metatarsals should be of equal length on the antero-posterior radiograph. The third, fourth, and fifth metatarsals should then decrease in length from this reference point by 3 mm, 6 mm, and 12 mm, respectively. All of the osteotomies are fixed by dedicated screws.

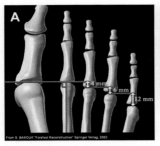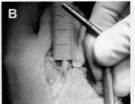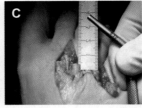

Fig. 6. Respect of the metatarsal formula (Besse, Maestro). (*A*) The metatarsal parabola. (*B, C*) Assessment of the relative lengths of the metatarsals, using the dorsal/proximal fragment to measure.

Additional procedures

This calculation may need to be adjusted intraoperatively as follows. On the first ray, the correction of the hallux valgus must be complete with the load simulation test [23]. On the lateral rays, the correction of the MTP dislocation, as well as any lateral deviation, must also be complete and without any tightness. This sometimes requires an additional shortening of 2 to 4 mm beyond what was calculated preoperatively (Fig. 5).

In addition, a hallux proximal phalangeal osteotomy is performed and fixed with dedicated staples [24,25]. On the lesser toes, a soft tissue release of the contracted tendons and ligaments responsible for the proximal interphalangeal flexion deformity is accomplished through an open incision [26]. Kirschner wires are used to temporarily hold the reduction of the realigned proximal interphalangeal joints for several weeks. The Kirschner wires do not cross the MTP joint. Lesser toe proximal interphalangeal joint fusion or resection arthroplasty is avoided in most cases.

In all cases, lengthening of the tendons was performed as required. However, in no case was a flexor-to-extensor tendon transfer performed or felt to be necessary. Because of the generally advanced stage of the rheumatoid disease, synovectomy of the MTP joints was rarely required. More commonly it was necessary to remove rheumatoid nodules from the plantar forefoot and digits. In five patients, a proximal gastrocnemius recession was performed as a separate procedure, generally 3 days before the foot procedure (Fig. 7) [27–29].

This surgery takes more time and is more technically demanding than the traditional first-MTP joint fusion and lateral metatarsal head resections. Notably, the metatarsal heads are often impaired. This can make the bony fixation fragile and require more time to heal (40 days in a heel support shoe). However, the results are such that the authors continue to perform rheumatoid forefoot reconstructions in this way.

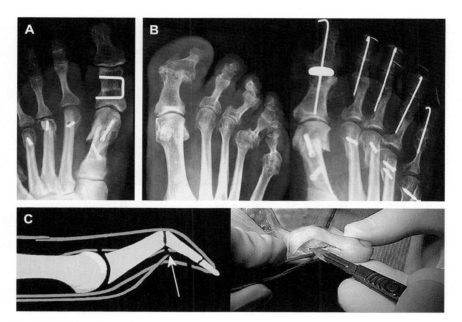

Fig. 7. Additional procedures. (*A*) Great toe proximal phalanx osteotomy. (*B*) "Button" prosthesis (temporary spacer) on the great toe interphalangeal joint. (*C*) Because the lateral toe joints are not affected by rheumatoid disease, they are generally preserved during surgery; only proximal interphalangeal plantar release and temporary K-wiring is necessary.

Nonpreservation joint surgery

On the first ray. In a severely impaired, arthritic hallux MTP joint, MTP arthrodesis is performed instead of joint preservation. This is achieved using dedicated "20" memory staples [30]. If the hallux interphalangeal joint is arthritic, an arthroplasty with a "button" prosthesis is performed [31].

On the lateral rays. When the lateral rays are severely impaired and arthritic at the MTP joint, a metatarsal head resection is undertaken instead of a joint-preserving Weil osteotomy.

However, in no way is joint preservation ever abandoned because of the severity of the hallux valgus deformity or the extent of the lesser MTP joint dislocations.

Postoperative protocol

Weight bearing in a heel support shoe is permitted the day following surgery [32,33]. Because of the fragility of the preserved metatarsal heads in the rheumatoid patient, the shoe must be worn for more than a month. During the month following the procedure, taping or strapping of the toes is performed, primarily on the lesser rays. After the bandages are

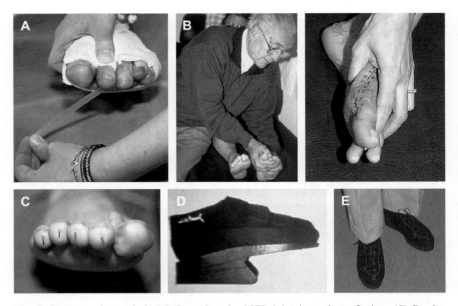

Fig. 8. Postoperative period. (*A*) Strapping the MTP joint into plantarflexion. (*B*) Passive mobilization, also in plantarflexion (the help of the husband is useful). (*C*) K-wiring for 1 month, excluding the MTP joint. (*D*) Our heel support shoe (type I) allows immediate walking recovery without any risk; however, patients have to wear it for 40 days because of the fragility of the preserved metatarsal heads. (*E*) Our variable volume shoe (type II) allows return to normal activities (both shoes made by Romans Industrie, France). (*From* Barouk LS. Forefoot reconstruction. 2nd edition. Berlin: Springer-Verlag; 2005. p. 389; with permission.)

discontinued, stretching and training of the toes is emphasized, most importantly plantar flexion of the MTP joints, for 2 to 3 months (Fig. 8).

Results

Results on the first ray

The results of correction of the hallux valgus deformity in this series were noted to be reliable and long lasting. With an average follow-up of 6 years and 3 months, maintenance of satisfactory correction was found in 95% of cases. The average range of motion of the first MTP joint at final follow-up was 55°. Contact between the great toe and the ground was well preserved with this procedure.

In our earlier experience with this technique, there were some cases of overcorrection with a resultant hallux varus deformity. This occurred because it is common to find in rheumatoid forefoot deformities a very wide hallux valgus angle with a contrastingly narrow intermetatarsal angle (average 13°). In these cases, the lateral translation of the Scarf osteotomy was too great, leaving a negative intermetatarsal angle, which led to the complication.

Impairment of the first metatarsophalangeal joint
and of the metatarsal head

Joint preservation of the first ray does not adversely affect the quality or condition of the first metatarsophalageal joint. On the contrary, it has been observed that generally the appearance of the joint improves, and this improvement is long lasting. Similarly, in most cases the condition of the first metatarsal head significantly improves radiographically with resolution of the cystic changes and peri-articular osteopenia associated with rheumatoid arthritis.

There was only one failure of joint preservation of the first ray out of the 55 cases performed in this series. This required revision to a first MTP joint arthrodesis. One spontaneous fusion of a first MTP joint following Scarf osteotomy was observed.

Primary first MTP joint fusion was performed in only 8% of cases. This was elected only when the MTP joint was arthritic or the bone quality of the metatarsal head was severely impaired.

On the hallux interphalangeal joint

When required, an arthroplasty of the first interphalangeal joint was performed with interposition of a metallic disk-shaped button implant

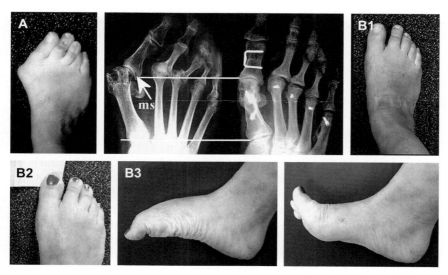

Fig. 9. Results on the first ray: preoperative and 4-year postoperative radiographs. Note the correction of the hallux valgus deformity and the improvement of the metatarsal head, with notable disappearance of the cysts, good MTP mobility, and preservation of toe-to-ground contact. (*From* Barouk LS. Forefoot reconstruction. 2nd edition. Berlin: Springer-Verlag; 2005. p. 389, with permission.)

in 15% of the cases in this series [7]. These buttons were removed at 1 year following implantation, after the inflammatory arthritis had subsided. Following this, the interphalangeal joint was relatively stiff but the clinical outcome was clearly better than that following fusion of this joint (Fig. 9).

Results on the lateral rays

Correction of the deformities

This study analyzed the relationship between the relative lengths of the lesser metatarsals and the clinical outcome. It was determined that any error in the final relative lengths of the metatarsals that deviated from the ideal metatarsal curve as described by Maestro and colleagues [22] led to secondary problems and failure of the procedure.

The results of the lateral ray procedures were also assessed individually, ray by ray, looking at maintenance of correction and percentage of metatarsal heads preserved. Complete correction of lesser MTP dislocation or subluxation was observed in 85% of the operated rays. There were no cases of complete recurrence of the dislocation noted following surgery. Partial subluxation of the lesser MTP joints was documented in 15% of the operated cases in this series. However, these patients did not report significant clinical symptoms from their recurrent deformities. These mild recurrent deformities were usually observed immediately after surgery. Revision was necessary in only one case.

These results were obtained with only Weil osteotomies and lengthening of the tendons as necessary. No flexor-to-extensor tendon transfers were performed in this series of patients. The hammertoe deformities were addressed with proximal interphalangeal joint plantar releases and temporary fixation with Kirschner wires. Only a few of the earliest cases in this series underwent proximal interphalangeal joint fusion.

On the lesser toes

The lesser toes contacted the ground during weight bearing in 85% of the operated cases, with the remaining 15% being "floating toes." In nearly all cases, the strength of the realigned lesser toes was relatively weak, but this was well tolerated in the low-demand rheumatoid population. Stiffness of the reconstructed lesser MTP joints was observed only in cases where the proximal sliding of the metatarsal osteotomy was insufficient, mostly in the earlier cases. Almost no stiffness was noted in cases where a large shortening of the metatarsals was achieved, especially when the amount of correction was focused on the MS point.

Recurrent or transfer metatarsalgia was observed in 10% of the operated lesser metatarsals. When symptomatic enough, these were successfully treated with a Barouk–Rippstein–Toullec (BRT) osteotomy (Fig. 11) [33–35].

Impairment of the lateral metatarsophalangeal joints
and of the metatarsal heads

Metatarsophalangeal joints. Because dislocation of the joint obscures the joint space on preoperative radiographs, the status of the articular surfaces of the MTP joints was primarily assessed by direct visualization intraoperatively. In the rare cases where there was not a frank dislocation of the joint preoperatively, it was noted that there was a significant radiologic improvement in the joint space following Weil shortening osteotomy.

Metatarsal heads. Following Weil shortening osteotomy and realignment of the MTP joints, it was observed that there was significant radiologic improvement of the metatarsal heads in 85% of the cases. Cysts within the head of the metatarsal disappeared over time and the normal trabecular appearance of the bone was restored (Fig. 10).

Primary lesser metatarsal head resection was performed in only 14% of cases due to severe impairment of the joint or head. Failed joint preservation of the lesser MTP joint resulting in secondary metatarsal head resection occurred in only 2% of the cases.

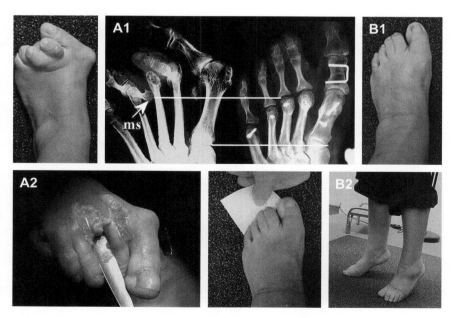

Fig. 10. Results on the lateral rays. Preoperative and 2.5-year postoperative radiographs. Note the correction of the MTP dislocation—whatever the grade—after Weil osteotomies, which respect the MS point. In spite of the large metatarsal shortening required, the global foot shortening is not very significant thanks to the preservation of toe length. Also apparent is the improvement of the corresponding metatarsal heads and the good functional outcomes. (*From* Barouk LS. Forefoot reconstruction. 2nd edition. Berlin: Springer-Verlag; 2005. p. 389, with permission.)

On the toes

The results of correction of toe deformities in this series must also be distinguished between early and later cases. Because lesser-toe proximal interphalangeal fusion and resection arthroplasty have been largely abandoned for the plantar proximal interphalangeal joint release procedure, there have been no major recurrences of toe deformity (Figs. 10 and 11).

Discussion

Degree of shortening: the MS point

The authors have observed that to obtain successful correction of the deformities and improvement of the metatarsal head and joint appearance, the shortening should reach the MS point of the most impaired ray. Undercorrected metatarsals lead to inadequate realignment and continued impairment of the joint. Overshortening of the metatarsals, on the contrary, can still provide good clinical results (Fig. 12).

Joint preservation

When discussing joint preservation in the rheumatoid forefoot, there are typically two clinical scenarios:

The first is a patient in whom the inflammatory period has resolved both clinically as well as by CT scan. By the time they present to the orthopaedic clinic, these patients usually have severe deformities due to the advanced stage of their disease. However, the deformity is considered a static condition. In other nonrheumatologic conditions where a severe static forefoot deformity is present, whatever its grade or origin (eg, advanced hallux valgus, iatrogenic deformity), the authors have observed that the large and harmonized shortening of all the metatarsals allows reliable correction of severe forefoot disorders. Naturally, the authors applied the same joint-preserving techniques to severe static rheumatoid forefeet and have found

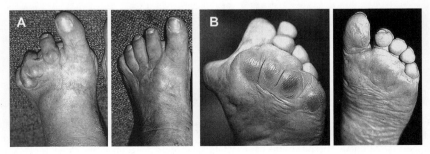

Fig. 11. Results on the lateral rays. Correction of severe claw toe deformity and metatarsalgia by large metatarsal shortening only. (*From* Barouk LS. Forefoot reconstruction. 2nd edition. Berlin: Springer-Verlag; 2005. p. 389, with permission.)

no difference in the results. That is, the corrections of the deformities have been good and long lasting.

The second clinical scenario is when the inflammatory period of the rheumatoid disease is still actively destroying or altering the joints of the forefoot. The shortening osteotomies are performed in the same fashion. However, the authors have observed that the inflammatory rheumatoid process tends to stop after this surgery (except in rare cases where the removal of rheumatoid nodules was necessary). The authors do not know the reason for this, but it may explain the long-lasting correction of the deformities and improvement in the appearance of the bone and MTP joint over time.

Lesser toes

The interphalangeal joints of the lesser toes may be very deformed, but they are not affected by the rheumatoid disease itself. Therefore, an interphalangeal joint fusion or resection arthroplasty is not necessary. The

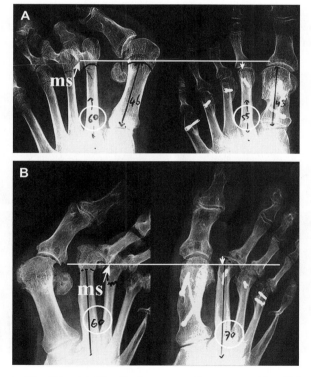

Fig. 12. Respect of the MS point. Usually, the preoperative assessment is sufficient, and respect of the calculated shortening assures a good result; however, what happens when we modify this assessment? (*A*) In this case, the metatarsal was shortened a few millimeters more intraoperatively than calculated, with no clinical consequences. (*B*) In this case, the metatarsal shortening was less than the preoperative assessment, a bad result. Therefore, the shortening assessed by the MS point may be slightly increased, but never decreased.

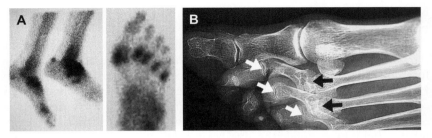

Fig. 13. Osteotomies are performed on the MTP joints, whereas only soft tissue releases are necessary in the proximal interphalangeal joints. (*A*) Bone scan of a rheumatoid forefoot showing increased uptake primarily at the MTP joints, which is the location of the rheumatoid lesions. (*B*) Plain films of the lesser toes with well-preserved proximal interphalangeal joints, which are typically not involved in the rheumatoid process.

authors have observed that a plantar release of the proximal interphalangeal joint combined with lengthening of the tendons is sufficient in most cases for correction of these deformities. Therefore, although the authors have shortened the metatarsals, the length of the toes has been maintained by preserving the interphalangeal joints (Figs. 12 and 13).

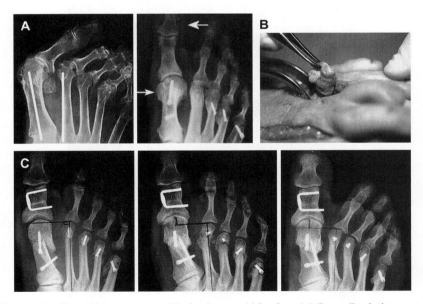

Fig. 14. Specific problems encountered in the rheumatoid forefoot. (*A*) Generally, the intermetatarsal angle is low (contrasting with a high hallux valgus angle). This can lead to overcorrection of hallux valgus, as observed in our early experience. (*B*) Rheumatoid nodules may appear secondarily, requiring removal. (*C*) The preserved metatarsal heads are fragile in the postoperative period, needing more time with the heel support shoe; otherwise, (same case, middle, and right), secondary displacement may occur, resulting in lateral deviation and metatarsal shortening. In this case, this results in a 1st metatarsal that is too long, requiring a secondary shortening as well.

Forefoot joint preservation is always preferable to fusion or resection, especially in rheumatoid patients, many of whom have undergone previous hindfoot fusions. In pursuing joint-preserving surgery, however, the authors knew it was critical to show clinical results that were better or at least equivalent to the traditional first MTP fusion combined with lesser metatarsal head resections. In fact, the functional results are better in most cases. Patients who have undergone joint-preserving surgery on one side and the traditional procedure on the other routinely prefer the side with the preserved joints. Other investigators have documented similar results [4–6].

Correction of deformity

On the first ray

One thing is clear from this study: First MTP joint preservation is possible thanks to extraarticular metatarsal shortening, which provides good and long-lasting correction of the hallux valgus deformity. This technique can replace traditional first MTP joint arthrodesis in almost all cases. It is important to take into account the narrow intermetatarsal angles typically seen in this rheumatoid patient group. By far the most critical component of the correction is shortening, with only a small lateral displacement of the osteotomy.

On the lateral rays

The metatarsal shortening obtained by the Weil osteotomy can correct most deformities, particularly MTP joint dislocation. The correction is also long lasting, so that in most cases it can replace traditional metatarsal head resection. It is remarkable that this correction is routinely obtained without the use of a tendon transfer, such as the Girdlestone–Taylor flexor-to-extensor procedure used notably by Rippstein [5]. This is due to the large amount of shortening that can be achieved by the Weil osteotomy, as well as to careful postoperative strapping of the toes. When impairment of the metatarsal head is extreme, metatarsal head resection is preferable.

Improvement of the metatarsophalangeal joints and reconstruction of the metatarsal heads

The authors cannot explain why this improvement occurs. It is simply an observation. However, the significant improvement of these structures reinforces the authors' interest in metatarsal and MTP-joint–preserving surgery in the rheumatoid forefoot (Figs. 9–10).

Global shortening of the foot

The shortening of the first ray following joint preservation is not significantly greater than the shortening following first MTP arthrodesis. Because of the severe impairment of the joint in patients who require fusion, a large amount of diseased bone often must be debrided to achieve a stable fusion. This results in significant shortening of the first ray following arthrodesis (average 7–10 mm). Shortening following joint-preserving Scarf osteotomy is typically 11 mm (7–15 mm).

On the lesser rays, the traditional metatarsal head resection removes about 10 mm of bone. The average shortening by a Weil osteotomy is 13 mm, but because the authors preserve the interphalangeal joint, this results in a similar overall shortening of the ray compared with head resection, which is generally combined with a proximal interphalangeal joint fusion or resection.

Respect of the metatarsal curve

The equal lengths of the first and second metatarsals during shortening must be absolutely respected. At most, the second metatarsal can be 2 mm longer than the first metatarsal, but the first metatarsal must never be longer than the second. This error can result in overload of the first ray, overcorrection of the hallux valgus, and no improvement in the quality of the first metatarsal head.

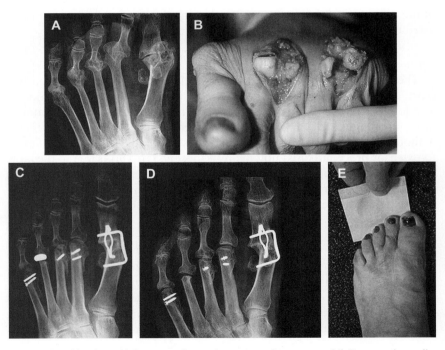

Fig. 15. Combination of joint-preserving and nonpreserving surgery. (A) Preoperative radiograph. Note the severe impairment of the 4th metatarsal head, which required a resection arthroplasty and a temporary spacer ("button"). Similarly we performed a 1st MTP fusion, but the other rays were preserved, and we noted the progressive improvement of the corresponding metatarsal heads and long-term good clinical result. (C, D) Four-year follow-up.

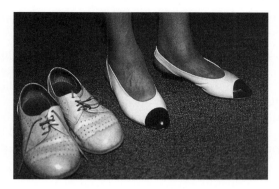

Fig. 16. Chanel shoes on a rheumatoid patient 1 year postoperatively. Rheumatoid patients also like to wear fashionable shoes!

Specific problems encountered in a rheumatoid forefoot

Technical problems encountered during joint-preservation surgery include excessive lateral translation of the Scarf osteotomy leading to overcorrection of the bunion. The narrow first intermetatarsal angle often seen in rheumatoid feet must be recognized, and a moderate translation should be performed to avoid a negative intermetatarsal angle. Other problems include the fragility of the retained metatarsal heads, which can lead to difficulty in obtaining stable fixation or early failure of fixation. Finally, with joint preservation, rheumatoid nodules may appear secondarily, which if symptomatic may require removal (Figs. 14).

Role of first metatarsophalangeal joint arthrodesis and lesser metatarsal head resection arthroplasty

First MTP joint arthrodesis and lesser metatarsal head resection arthroplasty are reserved for extremely impaired metatarsal heads and MTP joints. However, as the authors have noted, joint-sacrificing procedures can be combined with joint-preservation techniques within the same foot, depending upon the individual condition of each joint (Figs. 15,16).

Summary

The authors currently approach rheumatoid forefoot reconstruction with joint-preserving distal metatarsal osteotomies of all five rays. (The Weil osteotomy is distal by definition, and the Scarf because it includes a distal cut.) The authors do this because the main location of the rheumatoid disease in the forefoot is located at the MTP joint and metatarsal heads.

These osteotomies above all shorten the metatarsals, with two main consequences:

- They provide longitudinal decompression of the ray, which allows for reliable correction of any deformity with excellent results at long-term follow-up. These results are similar to those achieved following surgery for any other severe static forefoot disorder.
- They modify the local environment or conditions of the rheumatoid joint such that a significant improvement in both the MTP joint space and the condition of the metatarsal head can be observed.

However, only large amounts of metatarsal shortening focused on the MS point can provide reliable results; poor results are regularly observed when these conditions are not met. This surgery is definitely more technically demanding and requires more time to perform than the traditional one.

When the above conditions are satisfied, the correction is excellent and the results are long lasting (>13 years follow-up). There does not seem to be a limitation to the degree of deformity that can be corrected by this technique. The only limits of this joint-preservation surgery are the grade of the MTP joint arthritis and degree of metatarsal head impairment. Even moderate-to-severe impairment of these structures, when correctly addressed with the authors' procedure, can still potentially lead to preservation of the joint. Only extremely impaired joints or metatarsal heads should be considered for the traditional surgery (first MTP fusion and lesser metatarsal head resections).

In summary, excellent correction of the hallux valgus deformity in the rheumatoid forefoot can be achieved with a Scarf osteotomy in 92% of cases without the need for MTP joint arthrodesis. Similarly, 86% of the lateral metatarsal heads can be preserved using Weil osteotomies, with results similar or better than those for head resections. The authors continue to retain a role for the traditional surgery, but it is reserved for only extremely impaired rays. It is also acceptable to mix joint-preserving techniques with head resections in the same foot when necessary. Paralleling the recent improvements in the medical management of rheumatoid arthritis, joint-preserving surgery with Scarf and Weil osteotomies is a reliable procedure that marks a new direction in the surgical management of the rheumatoid forefoot.

Further readings

Barouk LS. Forefoot reconstruction. 2nd edition. (book and CD ROMs) Paris: Springer; 2005.
Barouk LS. Reconstruction de l'avant pied. (Book and CD ROMs) Paris: Springer; 2005 [in French].
Coughlin MJ. Rheumatoid forefoot reconstructon. A long term follow up study. J Bone Joint Surg Am 2000;(3):322–41.
Leemrijse T, Valtin B, Durez P. Avant pied rhumatoide. In: Chirurgie de l'avant pied. 2eme edition. Paris: Elsevier; 2005. p. 223–9 [in French].

Numez-Semper-Pizarroso M, Llanos Alcazar LF, Viladot Perice R. Technicas quirurgicas en cirurgia del pie. Barcelona (Spain): Masson; 2001 [in Spanish].
Regnauld B. The foot. Berlin: Springer Verlag; 1986. p. 87–101.
Barouk LS, Barouk P. Chirurgie du pied et de l'avant-pied. Available at: www.barouk-ls-p.com. Accessed July 28, 2007.

References

[1] Barouk LS. Correction des désordres statiques sévères de l'avant Pied par chirurgie extra articulaire:maîtrise orthopédique. Paris Gicep 2005;(No 144):6–21 [in French].
[2] Barouk LS. Severe forefoot disorders. In: Forefoot reconstruction. 2nd edition. Paris: Springer; 2005. p. 293–304.
[3] Maceira E. Osteotomias multiples instrumentadas en el Antepie para el Tratamiento de los sindromes de Insuficiencia del primer Radio. Clinica Osteoarticular 2001;4(n 1):7–14 [in Spanish].
[4] Hanyu T, Yamazaki H, Murasawa A, et al. Arthroplasty for rheumatoid forefoot deformities by a shortening oblique osteotomy. Clin Orthop Relat Res 1997;338:131–8.
[5] Rippstein P. Rheumatoid forefoot deformities. Surgical techniques in orthopedics and traumatology. Paris: Elsevier; 55-680-B-10; 2001. p. 1–5.
[6] Berg RP, Kelder W, Olsthoorn PGM, et al. Scarf and Weil osteotomies for correction of rheumatoid forefoot deformities: a review of 20 cases. Foot and Ankle Surgery 2007; 13(N 1):35–40.
[7] Barouk LS. Rheumatoid forefoot. In: Forefoot reconstruction. 2nd edition. Paris: Springer; 2005. p. 305–14.
[8] Barouk LS, Barouk P. Avant pied rhumatoide. In: Reconstruction de l'avant Pied. Paris: Springer; 2005.
[9] Barouk LS. Notre Expérience de l'Ostéotomie « scarf » des Premier et Cinquième Métatarsiens. Méd. Chir. Pied. Paris, Expansion Scientifique Française 1992;8(2):67–84 [in French].
[10] Barouk LS, Barouk P, Baudet B, et al. l'osteotomie Scarf du 1er Metatarsien et Osteotomie de la 1ere Phalange pour la correction de l'hallux Valgus. In: Valtin B, Leemrijse Th, editors. Chirurgie de l'avant Pied. Cahiers d'enseignement de la SOFCOT. Paris: Elsevier; 2005. p. 59–82 [in French].
[11] Barouk LS. Scarf osteotomy for hallux valgus correction. In: Myerson M, editor. Foot and ankle clinics, cracchiolo III A. Philadelphia: Saunders; 2000;vol. 5(n 3). p. 525–58.
[12] Borrelli AH, Weil LS. Modified scarf bunionectomy: our experience in more than 1,000 cases. J Foot Surg 1991;30:609.
[13] Rippstein P, Zund T. The scarf osteotomy for the correction of hallux valgus. Orthop Traumatol 2001;9:101–12.
[14] Weil LS. Scarf osteotomy for correction of hallux valgus. historical perspective, surgical technique and results. In: Foot and ankle clin. Philadelphia: Saunders; 2000;5(3). p. 559–80.
[15] Barouk P, Barouk LS. l'osteotomie de Weil du 1er metatarsien. In: Reconstruction de l'avant Pied. Paris: Springer; 2005. p. 11–114 [in French].
[16] Barouk P, Barouk LS. The Weil osteotomy of the first metatarsal. In: Forefoot reconstruction. Paris: Springer; 2005. p. 11–114.
[17] Barouk LS. The Weil lesser metatarsal osteotomy. In: Forefoot reconstruction. 2nd edition. a Book + CD ROMs. Paris: Springer; 2005. p. 115–38.
[18] Trnka HJ, Gebhard C, Muhlbauer M, et al. The Weil osteotomy for treatment of dislocated lesser metatarsophalangeal joints: good outcome in 21 patients with osteotomies. Acta Orthop Scand 2002;73(2):190–4.
[19] Leemrijse TH. Weil's osteotomy. Chirurgie de l'avant pied. In: Valtin B, Leemrijse TH, editors. Cahiers d'enseignement de la SOFCOT. Paris: Elsevier; 2005. p. 126–41 [in French].
[20] Barouk LS. The MS point. In: Forefoot reconstruction. 2nd edition. Paris: Springer; 2005. p. 60–65, 247, 291–338.

[21] Tanaka Y, Takakura Y, Kuma T, et al. Radiographic analysis of hallux valgus. J Bone Joint Surg Am 1995;77:205–13.
[22] Maestro M, Besse JL, Ragusa M, et al. Forefoot morphotype study and planning method for forefoot osteotomy. Foot Ankle Clin 2003;8:695–710.
[23] Kristen K. The load simulation test. In: Forefoot reconstruction. 2nd edition. Paris: Springer; 2005. p. 89.
[24] Barouk LS, Barouk P, Baudet B, et al. The great toe proximal phalanx osteotomy: the final step of the bunionectomy. Foot Ankle Clin N Am. Philadelphia: Elsevier; 2005;10. p. 141–55.
[25] Barouk LS. Hallux valgus. Proximal phalangeal osteotomy. In: Wulker N, Stephens M, editors. Atlas of foot and ankle surgery cracchiolo III.A. 2nd edition. London: Taylor & Francis; 2005. p. 1–7.
[26] Barouk LS. Hammer and claw toe of the lesser rays. In: Forefoot reconstruction. 2nd edition. Paris: Springer; 2005. p. 205–14.
[27] Barouk LS. Gastrocnemius proximal release. In: Forefoot reconstruction. 2nd edition. Paris: Springer; 2005. p. 158–67.
[28] Barouk LS. Gastrocnemius proximal release. In: Reconstruction de l'avant pied. Paris: Springer Verlag; 2005. p. 158–67 [in French].
[29] Barouk LS, Di Giovanni CH, directors. Proceedings of the symposium "Gastrocnemius tightness". SFMCP-AFCP French Spring Meeting Toulouse 2006 med Chir Pied. Paris: Springer; 2006;vol. 22. p. 131–58.
[30] Barouk LS. Use of the "20" memory staple in osteotomies and fusions of the forefoot. In: Forefoot reconstruction. 2nd edition: a book + 2CD rom. Paris: Springer; 2005. p. 168–73.
[31] Barouk LS. The button temporary spacer. In: Forefoot reconstruction. 2nd edition. Paris: Springer; 2005. p. 174–8.
[32] Barouk LS. Use of a post operative shoe without forefoot support, comparative study. Actualités en medicine et chirurgie du Pied, XVI 1986;57–69.
[33] Barouk LS. Post operative footwear. In: Forefoot reconstruction. 2nd edition. Paris: Springer; 2003. p. 91–3.
[34] Toullec E, Barouk LS, Rippstein P. Osteotomie de relevement basal BRT. In: Valtin B, Leemrijse Th, editors. Chirurgie de l'Avant Pied. 2eme edition. Paris: Elsevier; 2005. p. 142–8 [in French].
[35] Barouk LS. The BRT proximal metatarsal osteotomy. In: Forefoot reconstruction. 2nd edition. Paris: Springer; 2005. p. 205–14.

ELSEVIER SAUNDERS

Foot Ankle Clin N Am
12 (2007) 455–474

FOOT AND ANKLE CLINICS

Management of Hindfoot Disease in Rheumatoid Arthritis

Michael S. Aronow, MD[a],*,
Mariam Hakim-Zargar, MPH, MD[b]

[a]*Department of Orthopaedic Surgery, University of Connecticut Health Center Medical Arts and Research Building, 263 Farmington Avenue, Farmington, CT 06034-4037, USA*
[b]*Department of Orthopaedic Surgery, John Dempsey Hospital, Medical Arts and Research Building, 263 Farmington Avenue, Farmington, CT 06034-4037, USA*

The prevalence of rheumatoid arthritis in the United States is approximately 1%, which is higher than in other parts of the world [1]. Of 1000 patients who had rheumatoid arthritis, 89% had involvement of their feet, with the hindfoot and ankle involved in 66.9% and 8.8%, respectively [2]. The prevalence and degree of hindfoot involvement directly correlates with the duration of rheumatoid disease [2–5]. Patients who had less than 5 years of disease involvement had an 8% incidence of a disabling foot deformity as compared with 25% in those who had greater than 5 years of disease [6]. In another study, patients who had valgus hindfoot deformity had a longer mean disease duration (25 versus 14 years), more overall pain, and more forefoot pain than those who had normal alignment [7].

Some disorders, such as rheumatoid nodules, principally occur in patients who have rheumatoid arthritis. Patients who have rheumatoid arthritis can also develop the same hindfoot disorders as the general population, although not always with the same prevalence. Often the treatment is the same as for patients who do not have rheumatoid arthritis. Other times the expected progression of the disease process, the effect of rheumatoid arthritis on other parts of the body including the midfoot and forefoot, and the effects of the medications used to treat the disease can influence treatment recommendations.

Most patients who have rheumatoid hindfoot disease present with a history of the disease. Occasionally, however, undiagnosed patients present to a foot and ankle surgeon with symptoms and physical examination findings characteristic of rheumatoid arthritis or other systemic inflammatory

---

* Corresponding author.
E-mail address: aronow@nso.uchc.edu (M.S. Aronow).

1083-7515/07/$ - see front matter © 2007 Elsevier Inc. All rights reserved.
doi:10.1016/j.fcl.2007.05.003

disorders, such as multiple bilateral joint involvement, enthesopathy, or extensive tenosynovitis. In those situations, diagnostic laboratory studies may be ordered and the patient referred to a rheumatologist for confirmation of the diagnosis and medical management.

Clinical presentation and examination

As usual, a comprehensive history should be obtained and physical examination performed. Patients who have hindfoot involvement often complain of vague ankle pain and difficulty with ambulation. They also may localize their pain to more specific structural pathology and complain of weakness and joint stiffness.

The patient's neurovascular status should be evaluated. Pedal pulses should be palpated and the foot assessed for signs of adequate perfusion such as skin color, presence of hair, and nail condition. In addition to arterial insufficiency, vasculitis may be present and may also influence the surgical decision-making process with respect to timing, extent of surgery, risk for complications, and the need for vascular consultation. The presence of neuropathy should be evaluated using at least Semmes Weinstein 5.07 monofilament testing. Reduced protective sensation was noted in 59% of 51 patients and 28% of 25 patients who had rheumatoid arthritis [8,9]. Signs of Charcot arthropathy, such as a warm, erythematous, swollen foot, should be assessed. One should also attempt to elicit a positive Tinel's sign or modified Phalen's test to look for evidence of nerve entrapment, particularly tarsal tunnel syndrome [10].

The skin and subcutaneous tissues should be evaluated for callosities, ulceration, and rheumatoid nodules. Joint range of motion, swelling, and tenderness should be assessed. Tendon integrity, tenderness, swelling, contracture, and strength are evaluated. A Silfverskiöld test should be performed to assess for contracture of the gastrocnemius and Achilles tendon.

The bones of the hindfoot are evaluated for tenderness, exostoses, and deformity, including weightbearing hindfoot alignment and longitudinal arch integrity. Occasionally a cavovarus deformity may be present, particularly in patients who have juvenile-onset rheumatoid arthritis [11]. Pes planovalgus, however, is the most common hindfoot deformity in patients who have rheumatoid arthritis [2]. Over time, patients who have rheumatoid arthritis may develop progressive cartilage damage, capsular and ligamentous laxity, periarticular erosions, or tendon rupture leading to flexible or fixed subtalar joint pronation and lateral peritalar subluxation. The hindfoot valgus may be exacerbated by valgus tilt of the talus in the ankle mortise secondary to increased stress on a deltoid ligament already attenuated by the disease. Significant hindfoot valgus with subfibular impingement of the calcaneus may cause a fibular stress fracture [12]. Stress fractures may occur in other sites, including the distal tibia, calcaneus, and metatarsals. Tenderness over a Haglund's deformity of the posterosuperior calcaneal tuberosity may be seen in retrocalcaneal bursitis, insertional Achilles tendinopathy, and superficial calcaneal bursitis and over the plantar medial calcaneal tuberosity with plantar fasciitis.

Walking ability is assessed. Gait analysis studies in patients who have rheumatoid arthritis have demonstrated decreased walking speed and stride length and prolonged stance time [13,14]. In general, the degree of hindfoot disease has been associated with greater gait impairment than the degree of forefoot disease [14].

The ipsilateral hip and knee, contralateral lower extremity, upper extremities, and spine are assessed for abnormalities that may require treatment and influence the conservative or surgical treatment of the concurrent hindfoot pathology. Examples include upper extremity arthritis and weakness affecting the ability to maintain non-weightbearing status postoperatively and cervical spine instability, influencing the choices for anesthesia.

Radiographic evaluation

Weightbearing anteroposterior, oblique, and lateral foot, ankle mortise, and Cobey [15] tibiocalcaneal radiographs should be obtained to assess for arthritis, hindfoot alignment, and exostoses. If ankle or subtalar arthritis is a concern, then an anteroposterior ankle, Harris axial foot, and Broden's views may be added. If ankle instability is suspected, then mortise and lateral ankle stress views should be performed.

Additional bone and soft-tissue information can be obtained with MRI, CT, and ultrasonography. MRI is particularly helpful in assessing soft-tissue masses and tendon, ligament, and articular cartilage pathology. MRI criteria for synovitis and tenosynovitis are high signal intensity on T2-weighted images, low signal intensity on T1-weighted images, and Gd-DPTA enhancement in the joint or around the tendon [16]. Active synovitis appears hyperintense on fat-suppressed gadolinium T1-weighted spin echo images, whereas joint effusion appears hypointense on the same images [17]. One study, however, suggests a weak correlation between MRI and a rheumatologist's physical examination findings for hindfoot synovitis and tenosynovitis in 12 patients who had chronic polyarthritis, 9 of whom had rheumatoid arthritis [16]. Ultrasonography is operator-dependent but allows dynamic evaluation of tendons in a more cost-effective way than does MRI [18].

CT can be used to assess soft-tissue swelling, cartilage space narrowing, bony erosions, and pes planovalgus deformity as determined by increased heel valgus angulation, a tendency toward flattening of the sustentaculum tali, and medial and plantar slippage of the talar head [19].

Treatment overview

Soft-tissue disorders seen in the rheumatoid hindfoot include rheumatoid nodules, neuropathic ulcers, tarsal tunnel syndrome, plantar fasciitis, retrocalcaneal and superficial calcaneal bursitis, and tendon disorders, including tenosynovitis and posterior tibial tendon dysfunction. Bone and joint disorders include synovitis, arthritis, Charcot arthropathy, exostoses, and stress fractures.

The initial treatment of these disorders is almost always conservative. Optimal medical management of the rheumatoid disease process to limit inflammatory processes throughout the entire body including the foot is paramount and usually performed by a rheumatologist. Short-term cast or brace immobilization can be used in cases of acute inflammation. Various types of orthoses, braces, and shoe-wear modifications may be used for support and offloading. Physical therapy and home strengthening and stretching programs may provide symptomatic relief and maintain function. Selective corticosteroid injections may decrease local inflammation. In the presence of neuropathy, preventive foot care similar to that recommended for diabetic neuropathy should be practiced, including daily inspection of the feet and accommodative shoe-wear for ulceration and foreign objects, respectively.

Any patient who has rheumatoid arthritis undergoing surgery should have a thorough preoperative medical evaluation. If general anesthesia is being considered, clinical and, if indicated, radiologic assessment of the cervical spine should be performed including consideration of lateral flexion and extension views to assess atlantoaxial stability. In the absence of pedal pulses, vascular consultation and limited tourniquet use should be considered. Surgery should be delayed if possible in the presence of acute vasculitis. Because of the effect of the disease and the medications used to treat it, there is often atrophic skin and subcutaneous tissue present and an increased risk for wound dehiscence and infection [20]. Meticulous soft-tissue technique therefore should be used with sharp dissection where possible and gentle soft-tissue retraction. Because many rheumatologic medications, including methotrexate and Arava, are believed to inhibit wound healing, some surgeons have the patient discontinue them during the perioperative period. This may lead to exacerbation of the patient's systemic symptoms, however, and there is evidence that there is no increased rate of postoperative complications including infection and wound healing problems in patients who have rheumatoid arthritis who are taking nonsteroidal anti-inflammatory medications, corticosteroids, methotrexate, hydroxychloroquine, gold, and the tumor necrosis factor alpha inhibitors etanercept (Enbrel) and infliximab (Remicade) perioperatively [21,22].

Soft-tissue disorders

Rheumatoid nodules are firm, mobile masses containing chronic inflammatory cells and often a central area of necrosis [23]. They are found most commonly in patients who have long-standing disease in the subcutaneous tissues including overlying the Achilles tendon, the plantar heel pad, and bony prominences like the malleoli. They may be nontender or may cause symptoms from pressure with shoe-wear or weightbearing. With respect to treatment, optimizing medical disease management is important. Orthoses and various types of cushioned or donut-type pads can be used to avoid pressure on the nodule. There may be a role for injecting tumor necrosis factor alpha inhibitors into the nodules [4]. If symptoms persist, then surgical excision can be performed. If the lesion is on the plantar heel, care should be taken to avoid excessive resection of the adjacent plantar fat pad, and the plantar aspect of the nodule may need to be left in situ [24].

Neuropathic ulcers are initially treated with offloading and local wound care. Offloading may be performed with a total contact cast, a Charcot restraint orthotic walker (CROW), or a prefabricated diabetic walker. For plantar ulcers, weightbearing may be limited with crutches, a walker, or a wheelchair. Concurrent infection is managed with antibiotics and local wound debridement. Wound care options are beyond the scope of this article but include multiple types of dressings and wound-vac application. Surgical debridement may be required for deep infection. For recalcitrant ulceration, surgical excision of the ulcer with primary closure, flap coverage, or skin graft or skin substitute coverage may be considered. Bone prominences may need to be addressed with exostectomy, osteotomy, or fusion. A triceps surae contracture may require lengthening for ulcers at and distal to the level of Chopart's joints. Subcalcaneal ulcers, particularly those developing after excessive Achilles tendon lengthening, may benefit from a flexor hallucis longus to Achilles tendon transfer.

Tarsal tunnel syndrome is the most commonly seen nerve entrapment disorder [10]. Etiologies include tibial nerve traction from a hindfoot valgus deformity, compression from posterior tibial and long flexor tenosynovitis or other space-occupying lesions, the flexor retinaculum and deep fascia of the abductor hallucis, or tibial neuritis [3,4,11,25]. If there is a significant planovalgus deformity, an orthosis with medial hindfoot posting may decrease traction on the tibial nerve and its branches. A corticosteroid injection, anti-inflammatory medication, or a brief period of immobilization may decrease inflammation in the tarsal tunnel. Antineuritic medication such as gabapentin may be helpful. If symptoms persist, a tarsal tunnel release may be performed, including removal of any space-occupying lesions, such as tenosynovitis.

Plantar fasciitis is treated similarly to how it is in patients who do not have rheumatoid arthritis. Plantar fascia and triceps surae stretching exercises, cushioned shoe-wear with a heel cup or orthosis, rest, night splints, and local and systemic anti-inflammatory modalities, including ice, anti-inflammatory medication, and corticosteroid injections, are first- and second-line therapy. In recalcitrant cases, a period of cast immobilization or extracorporeal shock wave therapy may be helpful. Open or endoscopic partial release of the plantar fascia may be considered in symptomatic patients refractory to at least 6 to 12 months of appropriate treatment. It should be performed with hesitation, however, in patients who have significant fat pad atrophy or severe planovalgus deformities that may be exacerbated by partial loss of the windlass mechanism. In the latter, the gastrocnemius is usually contracted and a gastrocnemius recession with partial release of the soleus aponeurosis, if it is also contracted, may be more effective therapy.

Retrocalcaneal bursitis is initially treated with a heel lift, anti-inflammatory modalities and medication, and selective use of corticosteroid injections into the bursa. Superficial calcaneal bursitis is treated similarly with the addition of shoes with a soft or absent heel counter and consideration of an elastic brace with a silicone pad over the prominent "pump bump." Corticosteroid injections in the superficial calcaneal bursa should be performed only if the bursa is sufficiently large that it may be entered without injecting the Achilles tendon substance, which may increase the risk for tendon rupture, or subcutaneous fat, which may lead to atrophy and decreased padding. If either is recalcitrant, surgical excision of the bursa with excision of the associated bone prominence or Haglund's deformity and debridement of any associated Achilles tendinopathy may be performed.

Tenosynovitis may develop about the peroneal, posterior tibial, anterior tibial, and long toe flexor and extensor tendons and paratenonitis around the Achilles tendon. For mild to moderate tenosynovitis, anti-inflammatory medication and modalities, orthotic support, and physical therapy may be instituted. As extensive tenosynovitis may lead to tendinopathy or rupture, it should be treated fairly aggressively with a period of immobilization in a cast or cast walker. Although controversial, consideration of one corticosteroid injection in the tendon sheath may be considered, being careful to avoid injecting the tendon substance. If this is ineffective, an open or endoscopic tenosynovectomy can be performed, debriding or repairing any concurrent tendinosis or tendon tears [26]. For those less proficient in establishing tendoscopy portals, the addition of a 2.7-mm arthroscope and 2.9-mm or 3.5-mm full radius shaver to one or two limited open incisions can limit the amount of dissection needed to adequately evaluate the extent of tenosynovitis and subsequently debride it.

Complete tendon rupture may occur with the option of benign neglect versus surgical repair if diagnosed acutely. In the case of anterior tibial tendon rupture treated nonoperatively, an ankle foot orthosis (AFO) brace may improve gait by limiting foot slap on heel strike and dragging of the toes on swing phase. If noted nonacutely, the options are benign neglect with consideration of an AFO brace versus delayed surgical reconstruction. Usually the tendon ends have retracted and cannot be directly reapproximated. Occasionally, such as in chronic Achilles tendon ruptures, the gap in the over-lengthened tendon has been filled with scar tissue that may be partially excised, recreating appropriate tendon length and muscle tension. When a gap exists, it must be filled with an interposition graft or turndown flap or augmented with a tendon transfer. The interposition graft may be an autograft taken from half of one of the remaining tendon stumps or a distinct site, such as a toe extensor or a hamstring tendon, an allograft tendon, or a xenograft collagen-based tissue matrix product. With respect to specific tendon transfers, the flexor hallucis longus [27,28] is the most advantageous and commonly used for the Achilles tendon, with other options including the flexor digitorum longus [29] and peroneus brevis [30,31]. For the peroneal tendons, the peroneus brevis and the peroneus longus may be tenodesed together, or if both are torn with gaps at the same level, a flexor hallucis longus transfer to the peroneus brevis may be performed [32]. For the anterior tibial tendon, the extensor hallucis longus may be used [33], or for avulsions off of the insertion, the tendon may be reattached more proximally into the navicular using interference screws or suture anchors. The extensor hallucis longus and extensor digitorum longus may be tenodesed to each other. Chronic tears of the flexor hallucis longus and flexor digitorum longus are usually minimally symptomatic and not repaired.

Posterior tibial tendon dysfunction

In one study of 99 patients who had rheumatoid arthritis, 11% of patients had posterior tibial tendon dysfunction using stringent diagnostic criteria, including loss of the longitudinal arch, inability to perform a heel-rise, and lack of a palpable posterior tibial tendon [34]. In Johnson and Strom [35] stage I and II disease in which there is no deformity or a flexible planovalgus deformity, respectively, initial therapy consists of orthotic support. In mild deformity, a prefabricated or custom insole with medial hindfoot posting and medial longitudinal arch support or an elastic, stirrup, or lace-up ankle brace may be sufficient. If there is complete tendon rupture or more severe deformity, these devices may not provide sufficient support, and a custom University of California Biomechanics Laboratory (UCBL) brace, solid or hinged ankle foot orthosis, or Arizona brace may be required. Physical therapy consisting of triceps surae stretching exercises and foot and ankle strengthening exercises should be initiated [36]. Anti-inflammatory modalities, including ice, ultrasound, or iontophoresis, may be added. Corticosteroid injection into the tendon sheath may be associated with an increased risk for posterior tibial tendon rupture. There may be a fair amount of symptomatic relief afterward, however, and if the posterior tibial tendon is already ruptured or degenerated to the point that the next step is surgical excision, then the potential morbidity of an injection is minimal. Intra-articular corticosteroid injection may also provide symptomatic relief for associated subtalar arthritis or synovitis secondary to the anterior process of the calcaneus impinging against the lateral process of the talus. In stage III [35] fixed planovalgus deformities and stage IV [37] deformities in which there is also valgus deformity at the ankle joint secondary to arthritis or deltoid insufficiency, more commonly an ankle foot orthosis or Arizona Brace is required.

The surgical treatment of stage I posterior tibial tendon dysfunction is similar to that for non-rheumatoid arthritis patients. Posterior tibial tendon pathology is addressed with tenosynovectomy, debridement, repair, and augmentation as necessary. Augmentation is performed for significant tendinopathy or complete rupture and is usually performed using the flexor digitorum longus, with the flexor hallucis longus and peroneus brevis being less commonly used alternatives. Any pathology in the spring ligament complex is addressed by repair or imbrication and consideration can be made toward adding a gastrocnemius recession if a significant contracture is present. What constitutes a significant contracture and whether or not the advantages of decreasing the compensatory subtalar pronation and posterior tibial tendon strain associated with a triceps surae contracture outweigh the potential complications of gastrocnemius recession or tendo-Achilles lengthening is controversial and not adequately addressed in the literature. These potential complications can include calf weakness, wound problems including scar contracture, and sural nerve injury. The senior author's personal preference is to perform a gastrocnemius lengthening if after an adequate stretching program there is still less than neutral ankle dorsiflexion with the knee in extension and the talonavicular joint in neutral supination. The gastrocnemius aponeurosis is released through a small medial calf incision at the level of the gastrocnemius soleus interval. If the release is performed just distal to the level of the myotendinous junction, the aponeurosis is reattached to the soleus fascia at the appropriate length to limit weakness and improve cosmesis by having a less extensive proximal muscle bulge. If done more proximally, the gastrocnemius muscle superficial to its aponeurosis is left intact [38]. If after gastrocnemius lengthening has been performed there is still less than neutral ankle dorsiflexion with the knee in flexion, then a partial release of the soleus aponeurosis leaving the deeper soleus muscle fibers intact is performed through the same incision.

In stage II disease the same soft-tissue procedures are considered, although if there is less than −5° to −10° of ankle dorsiflexion with the knee flexed, a Hoke percutaneous tendo-Achilles lengthening is considered instead of a gastrocnemius recession. If there is minimal to mild arthritis by physical examination, plain radiographs, and, if still unclear, MRI or CT scan, a motion-sparing procedure to help restore the longitudinal arch and decrease strain on the posterior tibial tendon is performed. Potential procedures include medial displacement calcaneal osteotomy, Evan's intracalcaneal lengthening osteotomy, Cotton medial cuneiform dorsal opening wedge osteotomy, and subtalar arthroereisis. Other options include arthrodeses with limited effect on hindfoot motion such as naviculocuneiform and first tarsometatarsal joint fusion, and in the presence of calcaneocuboid joint arthritis, calcaneocuboid distraction arthrodesis. Given the potential progressive joint destruction seen in patients who have rheumatoid arthritis, a more significant motion limiting procedure, such as a subtalar, talonavicular, or triple arthrodesis, may be considered, particularly in the presence of decreased joint range of motion, arthritis, or moderate joint tenderness. For example, isolated talonavicular arthrodesis has been advocated in the flexible rheumatoid flatfoot to prevent the progression of hindfoot and forefoot deformities [39–41].

In stage III disease, a subtalar, talonavicular, double arthrodesis (talona-vicular and calcaneocuboid joints), or triple arthrodesis is usually per-formed. If there is less than neutral ankle dorsiflexion with the arch recreated nonweightbearing, a triceps surae lengthening procedure is consid-ered. A posterior tibial tendon debridement or augmentation is usually also performed with an isolated subtalar arthrodesis and may be considered with a double or triple arthrodeses if there is significant tendon tenderness.

In stage IV disease the procedures for stage II and III are performed with the addition of a deltoid ligament repair or reconstruction [42], ankle arthrod-esis, or ankle replacement arthroplasty. A deltoid ligament repair or recon-struction is considered when there is valgus tilt of the ankle secondary to deltoid insufficiency but with only mild ankle arthritis and lateral joint space narrowing. If moderate arthritis is present the procedure may still be consid-ered but with the addition of a medial displacement calcaneal osteotomy or a supramalleolar osteotomy to realign the ankle joint. A pantalar arthrodesis significantly restricts, if not eliminates, hindfoot motion and in the presence of ipsilateral hip, knee, midfoot, or forefoot arthritis can be functionally fairly limiting. With the presence of a shoe with a solid ankle cushion heel (SACH) and rocker bottom sole, however, motion during gait is not signifi-cantly different than with a rigid AFO or Arizona brace. The patient's re-sponse to bracing or a period of immobilization in a walking cast can be used as a trial to see if the patient tolerates the decreased motion after a pan-talar arthrodesis. If the Chopart's joints can be preserved, approximately 20° of hindfoot dorsiflexion/plantarflexion and supination/pronation motion can be maintained. Occasionally a motion sparing procedure can be performed in conjunction with an arthrodesis of only the ankle joint, thereby preserving hindfoot supination/pronation motion. Ankle replacement arthroplasty pre-serves ankle joint motion, which also decreases stress on adjacent joints. There is a higher complication rate, however, including the risk for implant failure requiring revision arthroplasty or implant removal and fusion [43,44].

Bone and joint disorders

Mild to moderate hindfoot synovitis and arthritis is treated with rest, or-thoses or braces, anti-inflammatory medications, physical therapy or a home exercise program, and corticosteroid injections. There may be a role for hyaluronic acid injections for moderate arthritis, particularly in the ankle joint. Not uncommonly, patients who have long-standing rheuma-toid arthritis may have significantly less pain than one would suspect by the extent of arthritis noted on examination and radiologic studies. Recalcitrant symptoms in the ankle or subtalar joint may require arthroscopic synovec-tomy, cheilectomy, and debridement of loose bodies and chondral flaps (Fig. 1). Talonavicular and less commonly calcaneocuboid pathology is most often addressed with an open incision, although arthroscopic approaches have been reported [45].

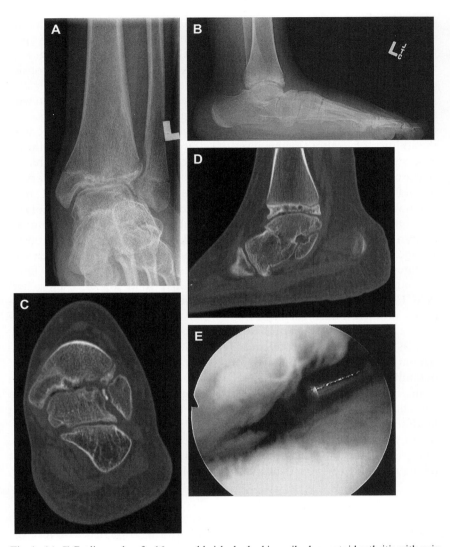

Fig. 1. (*A*, *B*) Radiographs of a 16-year-old girl who had juvenile rheumatoid arthritis with pain and crepitus principally overlying her anterior left ankle joint and greater than 20° of ankle motion. (*C*, *D*) CT scan images of the same patient. (*E*) Intraoperative ankle arthroscopy picture. Clinical improvement was noted after arthroscopic synovectomy, debridement of chondral flaps, and anterior tibial cheilectomy.

More severe arthritis of the hindfoot receives similar conservative treatment, although sometimes physical therapy may exacerbate symptoms by stressing the inflamed joints. Isolated subtalar arthritis is treated with a subtalar fusion. The procedure may be performed through an open [46] or arthroscopic [47] approach. With an arthroscopic approach usually only the posterior facet is denuded of cartilage and fused. For the open technique, a lateral incision from the distal aspect of the fibula extending anteriorly toward the fourth metatarsal base is made and the extensor digitorum brevis muscle retracted distally and dorsally to preserve its innervation and blood supply. Alternatively an oblique Ollier incision can be made. Fixation is usually obtained with one or two compression screws from the calcaneal tuberosity or dorsomedial talar neck. With good coaptation of the fusion surfaces and shingling or drilling of the subchondral bone, bone graft is generally not needed, although it is not unreasonable to add platelet-enriched plasma, local autograft, or demineralized bone matrix into the sinus tarsi area.

Isolated talonavicular arthritis without significant fixed hindfoot deformity may be treated with a talonavicular arthrodesis. A dorsomedial approach to the talonavicular joint is used. Fixation is usually obtained with compression screws or staples. External fixation is an alternative that may be more appropriate in the presence of acute infection or active Charcot arthropathy. Dowel autograft and allograft have been used [41,48] but are probably not needed with good coaptation and preparation of the fusion surfaces. Overall good results have been reported. In 31 patients, 26 who had rheumatoid arthritis, undergoing 35 isolated talonavicular fusions, 75% had complete pain relief and 89% had improved ambulation; however, 37% had progression of arthritis in other tarsal joints [39]. The same institution later reported on 104 patients who had rheumatoid arthritis who underwent isolated talonavicular arthrodesis with 95% good to excellent results and a 5% nonunion rate at mean 52-month (range, 1–16 year) follow-up with no known subsequent triple arthrodeses required [40,49]. In 19 isolated talonavicular fusions in 17 patients who had rheumatoid arthritis, there was a 63% union rate and good pain relief in all but 2 patients, one who had ankle arthritis and 1 in which the naviculocuneiform joint had initially been fused by mistake [41]. In 20 isolated talonavicular fusions in 19 patients who had inflammatory arthritis, 17 who had rheumatoid arthritis, there was a 95% union rate, good or excellent results in 19 feet, an average postoperative American Orthopaedic Foot and Ankle Society (AOFAS) Ankle-Hindfoot score of 89 (range, 35–97), and no change in hindfoot alignment during the average 37-month follow-up period [50].

Because there is little subtalar or calcaneocuboid joint motion after talonavicular fusion, some surgeons recommend additionally fusing the calcaneocuboid joint (double arthrodesis) [51], subtalar joint [52], or both (triple arthrodesis). Adding the additional joints to the fusion mass increases its stability, which would theoretically decrease the risk for symptomatic talonavicular nonunion. It would also eliminate the risk for another future operation and address unrecognized or subsequently developing arthritis in those joints. On the other hand, fusing these potentially asymptomatic joints involves potential increased morbidity caused by additional incisions, longer operative time, additional hardware that may require removal, and the risk for additional joints developing nonunion.

For patients who have fixed hindfoot valgus deformity and associated forefoot abduction and supination, triple arthrodesis remains the procedure of choice (Fig. 2) [53,54]. A standard lateral incision allows access to the subtalar, calcaneocuboid, and lateral talonavicular joints. A medial incision in the interval between the anterior tibial and posterior tibial tendons allows access to the remaining talonavicular joint. An approach through a single medial incision has also been described for patients who have poor quality lateral skin [55]. Fixation is obtained with compression screws or staples, with external fixation a good option in the presence of acute infection or active Charcot arthropathy. Again, with good coaptation and preparation of the fusion surfaces, bone graft is generally not needed, although it is not unreasonable to add platelet-enriched plasma, local autograft, or demineralized bone matrix into the sinus tarsi, calcaneonavicular, and medial talonavicular areas.

At average 5-year follow-up of 49 triple arthrodeses in 40 patients who had rheumatoid arthritis, 94% had significant pain relief, there was one symptomatic and one asymptomatic talonavicular pseudarthrosis, three patients had progressive ankle arthritis requiring pantalar arthrodesis, and there was no progression of ankle disease seen in patients whose hindfeet were corrected to 0° to 10° of valgus [53]. Of 132 primary triple arthrodeses performed with rigid screw fixation and average 5.7-year follow-up, 22 were in patients who had rheumatoid arthritis. The 22 rheumatoid feet all achieved union and required more correction than those that underwent the procedure for post-traumatic arthritis [56]. Solid and painless fusion was obtained in 93% of 282 patients who had rheumatic diseases who underwent 307 triple arthrodeses. The 21 failures, 18 of whom underwent successful revision surgery, were secondary to 14 malunions, 6 nonunions, and 1 painful foot without evidence of malunion or nonunion. Four of the malunions were secondary to progressive ankle disease and one case of avascular necrosis of the talus developed [54].

Advanced ankle arthritis can be treated with arthrodesis or arthroplasty. While allograft arthroplasty and distraction arthroplasty may have a role in nonrheumatoid patients, the progressive nature of the disease process, osteopenia, and immunosuppressive medications make them less appealing for patients with rheumatoid arthritis. Ankle arthrodesis in patients with rheumatoid arthritis has been performed through multiple different open [57–65] or arthroscopic techniques [66]. Clinical results have been variable with reported nonunion rates ranging from 60% [64] to 100% [66] in the above referenced studies. The senior author (Aronow, MS) prefers fibular sparing techniques to allow the option of future conversion to total ankle arthroplasty, to provide a buttress to prevent valgus collapse of the fusion, and to maintain the peroneal tendon groove and superior peroneal retinaculum. An arthroscopic approach, anterior approach, or lateral approach with a fibular osteotomy [59] can be used. An attempt is made to preserve length by maintaining the normal contour of the distal tibial and talar articular surfaces if possible. Fixation may be obtained with compression screws, blade plates, or external fixation. If the subtalar joint is already fused or

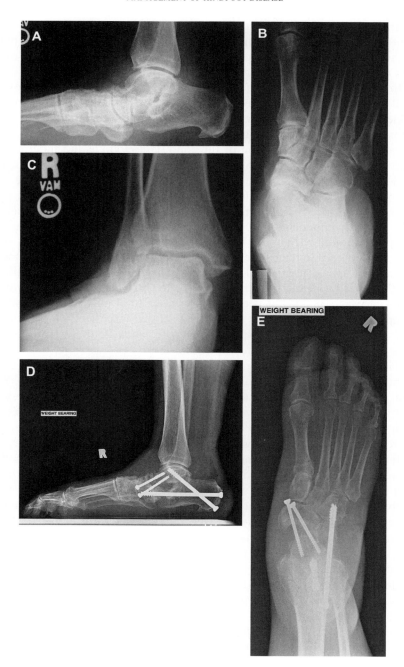

Fig. 2. (*A*, *B*) Radiographs of a 55-year-old woman who had rheumatoid arthritis and symptomatic posterior tibial tendon dysfunction unresponsive to conservative care. (*C–E*) Radiographs status post-triple arthrodesis and percutaneous Hoke tendo-Achilles lengthening.

arthritic, an intramedullary nail can be used, although the author prefers to limit this technique to cases with neuropathy due to the risk of lateral plantar nerve injury [67–68], or to cases with significant bone loss such as often seen after failed total ankle arthroplasty [43–44].

In some ways patients with rheumatoid arthritis are ideal candidates for total ankle arthroplasty while in other ways they are less ideal. The loss of ankle motion is less well tolerated and causes greater functional loss if there is ipsilateral arthritis or fusion of the subtalar, talonavicular, knee, and/or hip joints or decreased motion of the contralateral ankle and hindfoot. In a 20-year prospective study of 103 patients with rheumatoid arthritis, the ankle joint was usually affected only in patients with severe disease and was regularly preceded by subtalar pathology [69]. A subtalar fusion provides a larger base of support for the talar component and allows the use of stemmed components that may lead to a lower risk of subsidence and component failure (Fig. 3) [70]. Patients with rheumatoid arthritis also tend to be less active than patients with osteoarthritis and may have a shorter average life span potentially decreasing the incidence of component failure. On the other hand, there is a higher rate of complications including wound dehiscence and significant deep infection after total ankle arthroplasty as compared to fusion that may be poorly tolerated in patients with rheumatoid arthritis. There may also be more osteopenia in these patients and thus poorer support for the implants.

The intermediate-term results with first generation total ankle replacement in patients with rheumatoid arthritis were not very good [71–74]. Second generation implants, which in general are implanted without cement and are less constrained, have better short and intermediate term results with the majority of patients being satisfied with good clinical results and decreased pain [75–86]. However, the rate of significant complications including component loosening, wound dehiscence, and risk of amputation is much higher than for hip or knee implant arthroplasty. This may be in part related to the fact that second generation ankle arthroplasty is relatively early in its development and that there is a very steep learning curve in performing these surgeries. However, the poorer results may also be due to anatomical and biomechanical differences between the ankle and the hip and knee such as poorer soft tissue coverage and perfusion, increased force per unit area across the joint surfaces, and the complexity of balancing the ankle ligaments and aligning the bones and joints of the foot below [87]. Results are also greatly dependent on surgeon skill and experience along with the particular implant used.

Using the Japanese TNK implant in 19 patients (21 ankles) with rheumatoid arthritis, significant improvement was noted in pain score, range of motion, and walking ability at an average 34-month follow-up. There were two cases of delayed wound healing and one deep infection [78]. For 132 Agility implants with a mean 9 year (range 7–16 years) follow-up, 31 of which were implanted in patients with rheumatoid arthritis, there was

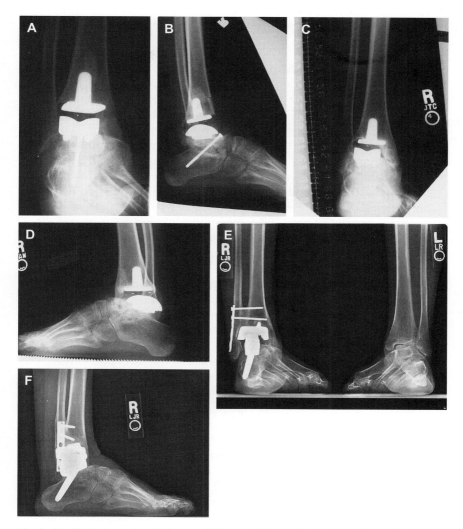

Fig. 3. (*A, B*) Radiographs of 15 year old female with juvenile rheumatoid arthritis seen for post-operative care after right subtalar fusion and ankle arthroplasty with Buechel-Pappas implants. (*C, D*) She subsequently underwent revision fusion of a subtalar nonunion at age 17 followed by hardware removal and ankle debridement at age 18. At age 19 she had persistent pain and functional limitations related to her ankle with x-rays as shown. (*E, F*) Radiographs 18 months after revision with custom Agility implant. She is currently pain-free and in her last year of nursing school.

an 11% revision or arthrodesis rate and a 76% incidence of peri-implant radiolucency. However, more than 90% of the surviving patients who retained their original implant reported decreased pain and were satisfied with their surgical outcome [84]. At average 3.3 year follow-up, all 10 patients with rheumatoid arthritis retained their Agility prostheses while 21 out of 52 patients with other diagnoses had underwent 17 revision arthroplasties, 2 conversions to arthrodesis, one conversion to an osteochondral allograft, and one amputation [88].

The Buechel-Pappas system has also been used in patients with rheumatoid arthritis [76,79–80]. In one study, 2 of 31 ankles had been converted to arthrodesis, one patient had passed away, and five ankles were interpreted as being at risk for impending failure because of marked tibial or talar component subsidence at an average follow-up of 8.3 years. However, 25 of the 28 remaining ankles had mild to no pain and were completely satisfied [79]. In another study with a mean 8 year follow-up, 15 out of 93 ankles required revision secondary to 6 cases of aseptic loosening, 6 cases of primary or secondary axial deformity with edge-loading, 2 deep infections, and one severe wound-healing problem. Perioperative complications consisted of 27 ankle fractures, 3 deep infections, and 8 wound-healing disturbances. Of the 57 surviving ankles, 48 had radiolucency around the tibial component and the mean AOFAS Hindfoot Ankle score was 77.0 as compared to 26.5 pre-operatively [76].

Several studies reporting on the results of the Scandinavian Total Ankle Replacement (STAR) have included patients with rheumatoid arthritis [75,77,81–83,85]. Using the original cemented version of the STAR prosthesis in 23 patients (27 ankles) with rheumatoid arthritis, there was noted to be significant improvement in pain, function, and mobility at one year postoperatively and a 75.5% implant survival rate at 6–14 years post surgery [82]. Another study evaluated 200 uncemented implants, 112 of which were placed in patients with rheumatoid arthritis. At mean 46-month follow-up, 146 had a good clinical and radiological outcome without any major complication and 14 patients had undergone revision or fusion. Major complications consisted of 5 major delays of wound healing, 19 perioperative malleolar fractures, 14 cases of established or threatened aseptic loosening, 9 cases of edge loading of the bearing surfaces, and 7 cases of pain and stiffness [81]. A different study evaluated 25 patients (28 ankles) with rheumatoid arthritis 3–8 years after uncemented STAR implantation. Six implants underwent revision between one and 51 months post-operatively. The remaining patients had an increase in their average Kofoed Score from 35 preoperatively to 71, and a final AOFAS Ankle-Hindfoot Score of 78.5 implants had a loose tibial and/or talar component. Overall, patients were satisfied with 18 of the STAR implants and not satisfied with 4 [83].

Summary

There is a wide variety of hindfoot disease seen in patients who have rheumatoid arthritis. Initial treatment is conservative, including optimizing medical management to control the disease process. Should symptoms persist, surgical treatment may be performed, although there is an increased rate of complications related to the disease and the side effects of the medications used to treat it.

References

[1] Alamanos Y, Voulgari PV, Drosos AA. Incidence and prevalence of rheumatoid arthritis, based on the 1987 American College of Rheumatology criteria: a systematic review. Semin Arthritis Rheum 2006;36(3):182–8.

[2] Vainio K. The rheumatoid foot; a clinical study with pathological and roentgenological comments. Ann Chir Gynaecol Fenn Suppl 1956;45(1):1–107.

[3] Cracchiolo A. Rheumatoid arthritis. Hindfoot disease. Clin Orthop Relat Res 1997;340: 58–68.

[4] Jaakkola JI, Mann RA. A review of rheumatoid arthritis affecting the foot and ankle. Foot Ankle Int 2004;25(12):866–74.

[5] Michelson J, Easley M, Wigley FM, et al. Foot and ankle problems in rheumatoid arthritis. Foot Ankle Int 1994;15(11):608–13.

[6] Spiegel TM, Spiegel JS. Rheumatoid arthritis in the foot and ankle—diagnosis, pathology, and treatment. The relationship between foot and ankle deformity and disease duration in 50 patients. Foot Ankle 1982;2(6):318–24.

[7] Keenan MA, Peabody TD, Gronley JK, et al. Valgus deformities of the feet and characteristics of gait in patients who have rheumatoid arthritis. J Bone Joint Surg Am 1991;73(2): 237–47.

[8] Wilson O, Kirwan JR. Measuring sensation in the feet of patients with rheumatoid arthritis. Musculoskeletal Care 2006;4(1):12–23.

[9] Rosenbaum D, Schmiegel A, Meermeier M, et al. Plantar sensitivity, foot loading and walking pain in rheumatoid arthritis. Rheumatology (Oxford) 2006;45(2):212–4.

[10] McGuigan L, Burke D, Fleming A. Tarsal tunnel syndrome and peripheral neuropathy in rheumatoid disease. Ann Rheum Dis 1983;42(2):128–31.

[11] Kitaoka HB. Rheumatoid hindfoot. Orthop Clin North Am 1989;20(4):593–604.

[12] Maenpaa H, Lehto MU, Belt EA. Stress fractures of the ankle and forefoot in patients with inflammatory arthritides. Foot Ankle Int 2002;23(9):833–7.

[13] Khazzam M, Long JT, Marks RM, et al. Kinematic changes of the foot and ankle in patients with systemic rheumatoid arthritis and forefoot deformity. J Orthop Res 2007;25(3):319–29.

[14] Platto MJ, O'Connell PG, Hicks JE, et al. The relationship of pain and deformity of the rheumatoid foot to gait and an index of functional ambulation. J Rheumatol 1991;18(1): 38–43.

[15] Cobey JC. Posterior roentgenogram of the foot. Clin Orthop Relat Res 1976;118:202–7.

[16] Maillefert JF, Dardel P, Cherasse A, et al. Magnetic resonance imaging in the assessment of synovial inflammation of the hindfoot in patients with rheumatoid arthritis and other polyarthritis. Eur J Radiol 2003;47(1):1–5.

[17] Boutry N, Flipo RM, Cotten A. MR imaging appearance of rheumatoid arthritis in the foot. Semin Musculoskelet Radiol 2005;9(3):199–209.

[18] Ostergaard M, Szkudlarek M. Imaging in rheumatoid arthritis—why MRI and ultrasonography can no longer be ignored. Scand J Rheumatol 2003;32(2):63–73.

[19] Seltzer SE, Weissman BN, Braunstein EM, et al. Computed tomography of the hindfoot with rheumatoid arthritis. Arthritis Rheum 1985;28(11):1234–42.

[20] Garner RW, Mowat AG, Hazleman BL. Post-operative wound healing in patients with rheumatoid arthritis. Ann Rheum Dis 1973;32(3):273–4.

[21] Bibbo C, Anderson RB, Davis WH, et al. The influence of rheumatoid chemotherapy, age, and presence of rheumatoid nodules on postoperative complications in rheumatoid foot and ankle surgery: analysis of 725 procedures in 104 patients [corrected]. Foot Ankle Int 2003; 24(1):40–4.

[22] Bibbo C, Goldberg FW. Infectious and healing complications after elective orthopaedic foot and ankle surgery during tumor necrosis factor-alpha inhibition therapy. Foot Ankle Int 2004;25(5):331–5.

[23] Arnold C. The management of rheumatoid nodules. Am J Orthop 1996;25(10):706–8.

[24] Shurnas PS, Coughlin MJ. Arthritic conditions of the foot. In: Coughlin MJ, Mann RA, Saltzman CL, editors. Surgery of the foot and ankle. 8th edition. Philadelphia: Mosby; 2007. p. 852.

[25] Cimino WG, O'Malley MJ. Rheumatoid arthritis of the ankle and hindfoot. Rheum Dis Clin North Am 1998;24(1):157–72.

[26] Bulstra GH, Olsthoorn PG, van Dijk NC. Tendoscopy of the posterior tibial tendon. Foot Ankle Clin 2006;11(2):421–7.

[27] Hansen ST. Trauma to the heel cord. In: Jahss MH, editor. Disorders of the foot and ankle: medical and surgical management. 2nd edition. Philadelphia: WB Saunders; 1991. p. 2355–60.

[28] Wapner KL, Pavlock GS, Hecht PJ, et al. Repair of chronic Achilles tendon rupture with flexor hallucis longus tendon transfer. Foot Ankle 1993;14(8):443–9.

[29] Mann RA, Holmes GB Jr, Seale KS, et al. Chronic rupture of the Achilles tendon: a new technique of repair. J Bone Joint Surg Am 1991;73(2):214–9.

[30] Teuffer AP. Traumatic rupture of the Achilles tendon. Reconstruction by transplant and graft using the lateral peroneus brevis. Orthop Clin North Am 1974;5(1):89–93.

[31] Turco VJ, Spinella AJ. Achilles tendon ruptures—peroneus brevis transfer. Foot Ankle 1987;7(4):253–9.

[32] Wapner KL, Taras JS, Lin SS, et al. Staged reconstruction for chronic rupture of both peroneal tendons using Hunter rod and flexor hallucis longus tendon transfer: a long-term followup study. Foot Ankle Int 2006;27(8):591–7.

[33] Mankey MG. Anterior tibial tendon ruptures. Foot Ankle Clin 1996;1(2):315–24.

[34] Michelson J, Easley M, Wigley FM, et al. Posterior tibial tendon dysfunction in rheumatoid arthritis. Foot Ankle Int 1995;16(3):156–61.

[35] Johnson KA, Strom DE. Tibialis posterior tendon dysfunction. Clin Orthop Relat Res 1989; 239:196–206.

[36] Alvarez RG, Marini A, Schmitt C, et al. Stage I and II posterior tibial tendon dysfunction treated by a structured nonoperative management protocol: an orthosis and exercise program. Foot Ankle Int 2006;27(1):2–8.

[37] Myerson MS. Adult acquired flatfoot deformity: treatment of dysfunction of the posterior tibial tendon. Instr Course Lect 1997;46:393–405.

[38] Blitz NM, Rush SM. The gastrocnemius intramuscular aponeurotic recession: a simplified method of gastrocnemius recession. J Foot Ankle Surg 2007;46(2):133–8.

[39] Elbar JE, Thomas WH, Weinfeld MS, et al. Talonavicular arthrodesis for rheumatoid arthritis of the hindfoot. Orthop Clin North Am 1976;7(4):821–6.

[40] Kindsfater K, Wilson MG, Thomas WH. Management of the rheumatoid hindfoot with special reference to talonavicular arthrodesis. Clin Orthop Relat Res 1997;340:69–74.

[41] Ljung P, Kaij J, Knutson K, et al. Talonavicular arthrodesis in the rheumatoid foot. Foot Ankle 1992;13(6):313–6.

[42] Bluman EM, Khazen G, Haraguchi N, et al. Minimally invasive deltoid ligament reconstruction: a comparison of three techniques. Presented at the 36th Annual Winter Meeting of the American Orthopaedic Foot & Ankle Society. Chicago (IL), March 25, 2006.

[43] Kotnis R, Pasapula C, Anwar F, et al. The management of failed ankle replacement. J Bone Joint Surg Br 2006;88(8):1039–47.

[44] Hopgood P, Kumar R, Wood PL. Ankle arthrodesis for failed total ankle replacement. J Bone Joint Surg Br 2006;88(8):1032–8.

[45] Oloff L, Schulhofer SD, Fanton G, et al. Arthroscopy of the calcaneocuboid and talonavicular joints. J Foot Ankle Surg 1996;35(2):101–8 [discussion: 186–7].

[46] Haskell A, Pfeiff C, Mann R. Subtalar joint arthrodesis using a single lag screw. Foot Ankle Int 2004;25(11):774–7.

[47] Tasto JP. Arthroscopy of the subtalar joint and arthroscopic subtalar arthrodesis. Instr Course Lect 2006;55:555–64.

[48] Thoren K, Ljung P, Pettersson H, et al. Comparison of talonavicular dowel arthrodesis utilizing autogenous bone versus defatted bank bone. Foot Ankle 1993;14(3):125–8.

[49] Dalziel R, Thornhill TS, Thomas WH. Isolated talonavicular fusion for hindfoot arthritis. Orthopaedic Transactions 1982;6:341.

[50] Chiodo CP, Martin T, Wilson MG. A technique for isolated arthrodesis for inflammatory arthritis of the talonavicular joint. Foot Ankle Int 2000;21(4):307–10.

[51] Mann RA, Beaman DN. Double arthrodesis in the adult. Clin Orthop Relat Res 1999;365:74–80.

[52] Sammarco VJ, Magur EG, Sammarco GJ, et al. Arthrodesis of the subtalar and talonavicular joints for correction of symptomatic hindfoot malalignment. Foot Ankle Int 2006;27(9):661–6.

[53] Figgie MP, O'Malley MJ, Ranawat C, et al. Triple arthrodesis in rheumatoid arthritis. Clin Orthop Relat Res 1993;292:250–4.

[54] Maenpaa H, Lehto MU, Belt EA. What went wrong in triple arthrodesis? An analysis of failures in 21 patients. Clin Orthop Relat Res 2001;391:218–23.

[55] Jeng CL, Vora AM, Myerson MS. The medial approach to triple arthrodesis. Indications and technique for management of rigid valgus deformities in high-risk patients. Foot Ankle Clin 2005;10(3):515–21.

[56] Pell RF 4th, Myerson MS, Schon LC. Clinical outcome after primary triple arthrodesis. J Bone Joint Surg Am 2000;82(1):47–57.

[57] Belt EA, Maenpaa H, Lehto MU. Outcome of ankle arthrodesis performed by dowel technique in patients with rheumatic disease. Foot Ankle Int 2001;22(8):666–9.

[58] Maenpaa H, Lehto MU, Belt EA. Why do ankle arthrodeses fail in patients with rheumatic disease? Foot Ankle Int 2001;22(5):403–8.

[59] Miehlke W, Gschwend N, Rippstein P, et al. Compression arthrodesis of the rheumatoid ankle and hindfoot. Clin Orthop Relat Res 1997;340:75–86.

[60] Dereymaeker GP, Van Eygen P, Driesen R, et al. Tibiotalar arthrodesis in the rheumatoid foot. Clin Orthop Relat Res 1998;349:43–7.

[61] Cracchiolo A, Cimino WR, Lian G. Arthrodesis of the ankle in patients who have rheumatoid arthritis. J Bone Joint Surg Am 1992;74(6):903–9.

[62] Felix NA, Kitaoka HB. Ankle arthrodesis in patients with rheumatoid arthritis. Clin Orthop Relat Res 1998;349:58–64.

[63] Anderson T, Maxander P, Rydholm U, et al. Ankle arthrodesis by compression screws in rheumatoid arthritis: primary nonunion in 9/35 patients. Acta Orthop 2005;76(6):884–90.

[64] Moran CG, Pinder IM, Smith SR. Ankle arthrodesis in rheumatoid arthritis: 30 cases followed for 5 years. Acta Orthop Scand 1991;62(6):538–43.

[65] Kennedy JG, Harty JA, Casey K, et al. Outcome after single technique ankle arthrodesis in patients with rheumatoid arthritis. Clin Orthop Relat Res 2003;412:131–8.

[66] Turan I, Wredmark T, Fellander-Tsai L. Arthroscopic ankle arthrodesis in rheumatoid arthritis. Clin Orthop Relat Res 1995;320:110–4.

[67] McGarvey WC, Trevino SG, Baxter DE, et al. Tibiotalocalcaneal arthrodesis: anatomic and technical considerations. Foot Ankle Int 1998;19(6):363–9.

[68] Pochatko DJ, Smith JW, Phillips RA, et al. Anatomic structures at risk: combined subtalar and ankle arthrodesis with a retrograde intramedullary rod. Foot Ankle Int 1995;16(9):542–7.

[69] Belt EA, Kaarela K, Maenpaa H, et al. Relationship of ankle joint involvement with subtalar destruction in patients with rheumatoid arthritis. A 20-year follow-up study. Joint Bone Spine 2001;68(2):154–7.

[70] Alvine GS, Steck JK, Alvine F. Early Results for the Agility Stemmed Talar Revisional Component for Total Ankle Arthroplasty. Paper presented at the 22nd annual summer meeting of the American Orthopaedic Foot & Ankle Society. La Jolla, CA: July 14, 2005.
[71] Hamblen DL. Can the ankle joint be replaced? J Bone Joint Surg Br 1985;67(5):689–90.
[72] Bolton-Maggs BG, Sudlow RA, Freeman MA. Total ankle arthroplasty. A long-term review of the London Hospital experience. J Bone Joint Surg Br 1985;67(5):785–90.
[73] Kitaoka HB, Patzer GL. Clinical results of the Mayo total ankle arthroplasty. J Bone Joint Surg Am 1996;78(11):1658–64.
[74] Unger AS, Inglis AE, Mow CS, et al. Total ankle arthroplasty in rheumatoid arthritis: a long-term follow-up study. Foot Ankle 1988;8(4):173–9.
[75] Carlsson A, Markusson P, Sundberg M. Radiostereometric analysis of the double-coated STAR total ankle prosthesis: a 3-5 year follow-up of 5 cases with rheumatoid arthritis and 5 cases with osteoarthrosis. Acta Orthop 2005;76(4):573–9.
[76] Doets HC, Brand R, Nelissen RG. Total ankle arthroplasty in inflammatory joint disease with use of two mobile-bearing designs. J Bone Joint Surg Am 2006;88(6):1272–84.
[77] Lodhi Y, McKenna J, Herron M, et al. Total ankle replacement. Ir Med J 2004;97(4):104–5.
[78] Nagashima M, Takahashi H, Kakumoto S, et al. Total ankle arthroplasty for deformity of the foot in patients with rheumatoid arthritis using the TNK ankle system: clinical results of 21 cases. Mod Rheumatol 2004;14(1):48–53.
[79] San Giovanni TP, Keblish DJ, Thomas WH, et al. Eight-year results of a minimally constrained total ankle arthroplasty. Foot Ankle Int 2006;27(6):418–26.
[80] Su EP, Kahn B, Figgie MP. Total ankle replacement in patients with rheumatoid arthritis. Clin Orthop Relat Res 2004;424:32–8.
[81] Wood PL, Deakin S. Total ankle replacement. The results in 200 ankles. J Bone Joint Surg Br 2003;85(3):334–41.
[82] Kofoed H, Sorensen TS. Ankle arthroplasty for rheumatoid arthritis and osteoarthritis: prospective long-term study of cemented replacements. J Bone Joint Surg Br 1998;80(2):328–32.
[83] Anderson T, Montgomery F, Carlsson A. Uncemented STAR total ankle prostheses. Three to eight-year follow-up of fifty-one consecutive ankles. J Bone Joint Surg Am 2003;85-A(7): 1321–9.
[84] Knecht SI, Estin M, Callaghan JJ, et al. The Agility total ankle arthroplasty. Seven to sixteen-year follow-up. J Bone Joint Surg Am 2004;86-A(6):1161–71.
[85] Kofoed H, Lundberg-Jensen A. Ankle arthroplasty in patients younger and older than 50 years: a prospective series with long-term follow-up. Foot Ankle Int 1999;20(8):501–6.
[86] Buechel FF Sr, Buechel FF Jr, Pappas MJ. Twenty-year evaluation of cementless mobile-bearing total ankle replacements. Clin Orthop Relat Res 2004;424:19–26.
[87] Gill LH. Challenges in total ankle arthroplasty. Foot Ankle Int 2004;25(4):195–207.
[88] Hurowitz EJ, Gould JS, Fleisig GS, et al. Outcome analysis of agility total ankle replacement with prior adjunctive procedures: two to six year followup. Foot Ankle Int 2007;28(3): 308–12.

ELSEVIER
SAUNDERS

Foot Ankle Clin N Am
12 (2007) 475–495

FOOT AND
ANKLE CLINICS

Ankle Arthrodesis in Rheumatoid Arthritis: Techniques, Results, and Complications

Vincent James Sammarco, MD

*Cincinnati Sports Medicine and Orthopaedic Center, 10663 Montgomery Road,
Cincinnati, OH 45242, USA*

Ankle disease in the patient who has rheumatoid arthritis (RA) typically develops as a complication of malalignment of the hindfoot or less often occurs without deformity, caused by destruction of the articular cartilage alone from the autoimmune process. Arthrodesis of the ankle can be fraught with complications if the surgery is not well planned, and special consider-ations must be given in planning the surgery to avoid postoperative problems. Primary fusion rates following ankle arthrodesis in patients who have RA vary in reports from 65% to 96%, averaging approximately 85%. Technical considerations for successful surgery must account for the increased surgical risks and challenges associated with RA. This article defines specific risks associated with RA, including an increased incidence of medical comorbidities, the use of steroids and other immunosuppressive agents, osteoporosis, vascular disease, and the common occurrence of severe deformity. This article suggests approaches for management and techniques that may improve specific surgical issues in this challenging patient population.

RA commonly affects the foot and may be the presenting feature of this disease process in 15% to 20% of cases [1,2]. Prevalence of ankle arthritis in patients who have documented RA is reported to be between 9% and 70% [3]. Although forefoot and hindfoot disease and deformity are common, primary inflammatory involvement of the ankle joint is less likely [4,5]. The disease process is mediated by an autoimmune process that is believed to be caused by an inappropriate activation of T cells and creation of autoantibodies. This in turn leads to the painful joint and tendon synovitis associated with the disease. Foot and ankle disease was divided into four

---

E-mail address: vjsammarco@csmoc.com

1083-7515/07/$ - see front matter © 2007 Elsevier Inc. All rights reserved.
doi:10.1016/j.fcl.2007.04.002

stages by Thompson and Mann (Fig. 1) [6]. Stage 1 involves synovitis without bony deformity or radiographic changes. In stage 2, involvement is more significant but without fixed or bony deformity. Radiographs may show erosive changes in the joint spaces. Synovectomy may be indicated if the synovitis is not controlled with medication. Stage 3 involves deformity caused by soft-tissue breakdown, and surgical reconstruction of supportive structures may be indicated to restore alignment. Stage 4 involves articular destruction, loss of cartilage, and often significant deformity. Surgery in the fourth stage of RA in the ankle is typically limited to arthrodesis or arthroplasty.

Ankle disease in the patient who has RA typically develops as a complication of malalignment of the hindfoot or less often occurs without deformity caused by destruction of the articular cartilage alone from the autoimmune process. Nassar and Cracchiolo [7] identified four issues associated with RA that lead to an increased risk for complications in these patients. Patients have systemic disease that affects not only the involved joint, but also causes degenerative changes of other organ systems. Patients who have RA frequently have other medical problems, such as diabetes, renal failure, and peripheral vascular disease, that further impair their ability to

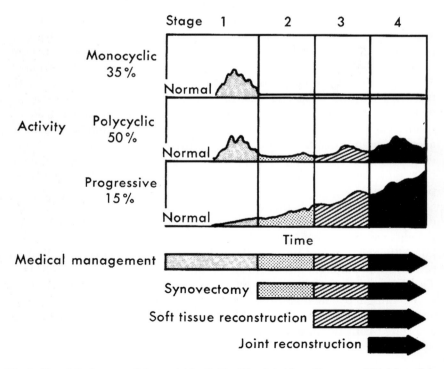

Fig. 1. The clinical course of rheumatoid arthritis. (*Reprinted from* Thompson FM, Mann RA. Arthritides. In: Mann RA, Coughlin MJ, editors. Surgery of the foot and ankle. 6th edition. St. Louis (MO): Mosby; 1993. Figs. 14–26, p. 646; with permission.)

heal these operations. The medications used to treat RA have effects that impair wound and bone healing. The patients may require multiple operations, and deformities tend to be advanced, requiring extensive and complicated surgery.

Considerations in medical management

Patients who have RA tend to have multiple joints involved with the disease process and also may have other medical issues not necessarily associated with inflammatory arthropathy. Involvement of an internist or the patient's primary care physician is important in preoperative planning, in hospital management, and in postoperative care. Patients who have coexistent diabetes need adequate control of blood sugars. In patients who have renal failure, dialysis must be arranged to coincide with the surgical schedule. Heparin should be held if surgery is within 36 hours of dialysis and may be held the following day or two as needed, depending on the amount of postoperative bleeding. Preoperative cardiac clearance is often necessary, because patients may have rheumatoid-related cardiac disease [8–10]. In longer-standing cases, rheumatoid cervical spine disease should be given some consideration, because anesthetic manipulation can cause paralysis if cervical instability is present [11–13]. Flexion and extension views can aid in diagnosing instability preoperatively [13].

Adjustment of the patient's medications in the perioperative period is important in maximizing the chances of successful surgery and also in decreasing the incidence of wound and bone-healing complications. Consideration should be given to stopping or decreasing the use of nonsteroidal anti-inflammatory drugs (NSAIDs), corticosteroids, methotrexate, and other disease-modifying agents. Discontinuation of these medications, however, can significantly affect the underlying rheumatic process and may cause recurrence of symptoms in other joints. The involvement of the patient's rheumatologist is important in achieving a balance between disease control and maximizing the patient's biologic potential for healing. Although few evidence-based guidelines exist for perioperative medication management, a summary with specific recommendations was recently written by Howe and colleagues (Table 1) [14].

Discharge planning is also of significant importance for these patients. Often patients have multiple joints involved that may make compliance with nonweightbearing restrictions difficult or impossible in the home setting. Most patients who have significant involvement of the upper extremities or contralateral leg require a stay in a subacute or acute rehabilitation facility.

Soft-tissue disease

RA is associated with deficiencies in the soft-tissue envelope that may lead to significant complications in wound healing. These deficiencies are

Table 1
Current recommendations for the use of antirheumatic medications in the perioperative period

Medication	Important drug interactions	Comments
NSAIDs	If using COX-2 agents for postoperative pain, consult a pharmacist. May affect function of antihypertensive agents and increase INR in older patients taking warfarin.	Discontinue five half-lives before surgery. Aspirin should be stopped 7–10 days before surgery.
Corticosteroids	Corticosteroid use with fluoroquinolones increases the risk for tendon rupture. Antifungal agents and clarithromycin may increase levels of corticosteroids.	Perioperative use depends on level of potential surgical stress.
Methotrexate	Methotrexate along with intravenous penicillins may lead to neutropenia.	Continue perioperatively for all procedures. Consider withholding 1–2 doses of methotrexate for patients who have poorly controlled diabetes, the elderly, and those who have liver, kidney, or lung disease who are undergoing moderate or intensive procedures.
Leflunomide	Leflunomide may elevate levels of warfarin and rifampin.	Continue for minor procedures, withhold 1–2 days before moderate and intensive procedures, and restart 1–2 weeks later.
Sulfasalazine	Sulfasalazine may increase INR in patients on warfarin.	Continue for all procedures.
Hydroxychloroquine	None	Continue for all procedures.
TNF antagonists	Avoid live vaccines in patients taking these agents; otherwise, no significant perioperative drug–drug interactions.	Continue for minor procedures. For moderate to intensive procedures, withhold etanercept for 1 week and plan surgery for the end of the dosing interval for adalimumab and infliximab. Restart 10–14 days postoperatively.
IL-1 antagonist	None	Continue for minor procedures. Withhold 1–2 days before surgery and restart 10 days postoperatively for moderate to intensive procedures.

(*From* Howe CR, Gardner GC, Kadel NJ. Perioperative medication management for the patient with rheumatoid arthritis. J Am Acad Orthop Surg 2006;14:545; with permission. Copyright © 2006 American Academy of Orthopedic Surgeons.)

related to the disease process itself, but also to the medications used to treat the disease. RA is associated with multiple skin manifestations that may alter the integument's ability to heal a surgical wound [15]. In addition, chronic glucocorticoid use decreases the structural integrity of the skin and subcutaneous tissues. Layered closures may be tenuous at best, because periosteum and the normal retinacular and muscular layers around the ankle are often atrophic and may not hold sutures well.

Chronic RA-associated vasculitis can also cause significant peripheral vascular disease and makes the vessels friable and susceptible to injury from minor mechanical trauma as may occur during surgery [16]. Patients who have RA also have increased risk for arterial vasospasm and arterial calcification [17]. In the event of limb ischemia during or following the surgery, arterial reconstruction is often not possible and may lead to amputation; therefore it is of critical importance not to perform major correction without enough bony resection to de-tension the soft-tissue envelope and vessels. The author routinely checks patients who have noninvasive vascular testing before surgery to ensure adequate blood flow is present to the extremity. Arteriogram and preoperative consultation with a vascular surgeon may be necessary if significant arterial disease is present. Poor vascularity of the extremity is a contraindication to surgery if arterial reconstruction is not possible.

Tendons may have significant degeneration and synovitis present. Rheumatoid nodules and exuberant synovium of the tendons and ankle joint should be excised to decrease the tension on the soft-tissue envelope during closure. Consideration can also be given to excising nonfunctioning tendons if needed to decrease soft-tissue tension during closure [18]. The combination of impaired vascularity and poor softtissue envelope quality makes final positioning and surgical techniques of the arthrodesis important. This has led some investigators to recommend a lateral, transfibular approach be used for patients who have RA, because it affords protection of the anterior and posterior neurovascular bundles while affording excellent exposure [19]. Significant deformity correction can place increased strain on the skin and vessels, which may be poorly tolerant of tension. Planning of the surgery should place the incision and approach on the side of the deformity that will not be under tension or the surgeon should plan on incorporating enough bony resection in the arthrodesis to allow for a tension-free closure.

Osteoporosis

Osteoporosis is present almost universally in RA and can cause significant complications when attempting to achieve stable arthrodesis with internal or external fixation [20]. Bone loss is present because of increased levels of circulating cytokines, such as tumor necrosis factor alpha (TNFα), interleukin (IL) 1, and IL6, which are present because of the chronic inflammatory process [21]. The exact pathophysiology of glucocorticoid-induced osteoporosis seems to be multifold, but it is well documented that higher doses and longer length of therapy are associated with increasing effect [22]. Methotrexate is also associated with catabolic bone loss [23]. A significant part of the etiology may be simply caused by disuse osteoporosis, because the patients may be limited in the amount of ambulation of which they are capable.

The severe osteoporosis associated with RA is often responsible for technical difficulties and complications during and after surgery. The metaphyseal bone of the distal tibia is often significantly affected and may have poor mechanical properties. The talus and the distal tibia may have areas of avascular necrosis caused by chronic steroid use that can further complicate the procedure [24]. The most common intraoperative complication is poor quality fixation caused by osteoporosis. This can lead to an unstable construct, recurrence of preoperative deformity in the postoperative period, cut out of the fixation, and failure of arthrodesis.

Problems with standard fixation techniques such as lagged screws have led to the development of fixation techniques that achieve more rigid fixation in poor quality bone. Some investigators have suggested primary tibiotalocalcaneal arthrodesis in patients who have RA, citing high nonunion rates in patients in whom compression screws alone are used [25–28]. Other investigators have recommended isolated tibiotalar arthrodesis be performed with more rigid fixation techniques. The use of a compression blade plate gives significant improvement in mechanical fixation during ankle arthrodesis and seems particularly suited to osteoporotic bone [29]. As locked plating technology has become available, fixation with these devices seems to offer distinct advantages in achieving a stable construct [30–32]. Other investigators advocate the use of a fibular onlay graft to improve fixation and stability in osteoporotic bone [29,33,34].

Clinical results

Ankle arthrodesis remains the gold standard treatment for end-stage ankle arthritis from rheumatic disease. Although achieving a stable arthrodesis can be challenging, durable deformity correction and pain relief can be expected once arthrodesis is achieved [35]. Several series note RA as a significant risk factor for nonunion of ankle arthrodesis. Various techniques have been reported with varying success at achieving arthrodesis in patients who have RA.

Compression screws

A common technique used for ankle arthrodesis in osteoarthritis and post-traumatic arthritis is joint resection and compression with larger diameter bone screws [36–39]. This technique has been shown to give worse results in some series in patients who have RA. Holt and colleagues [40] reported 23 cases of ankle arthrodesis and noted an overall fusion rate of only 74%; however, when higher-risk patients were excluded, the primary fusion rate increased to 93%. Anderson and colleagues [25] reviewed 35 open and percutaneous ankle arthrodeses in patients who had RA using cannulated screws for fixation. These investigators noted a 26% primary nonunion rate with no difference between percutaneous and open techniques. Only 57% of the patients were satisfied with the results, leading the investigators to conclude that ankle arthrodesis with compression screws did not give acceptable results in fusion rate or in patient function. Cracchiolo and colleagues [41] reported a 23% nonunion rate in 13 patients who had RA undergoing ankle fusion by internal fixation with compression screws, although function was reportedly good in those achieving stable arthrodesis in good position. Malunion in valgus was a problem in 2 of 13 patients and patients taking higher doses of steroids were at higher risk for infection and nonunion. Successful arthrodesis in patients who have RA has also been reported using absorbable fixation devices [42].

Arthroscopic fusion

Arthroscopic ankle fusion is appealing in patients who have RA, because this may protect the soft-tissue envelope more than an extensile approach [43–50]. The technique essentially involves excision of the joint surfaces and remaining cartilage with shavers and burs. Once the cartilage is removed, the subchondral bone is breached to the underlying cancellous surface and fixation, typically cannulated screws, is applied percutaneously under fluoroscopic guidance. The technique is limited in that significant rotational or varus/valgus deformity cannot be adequately corrected [51]. A significant learning curve is present [52,53]. Turna and colleagues [54] reported on 10 arthroscopic ankle arthrodeses in 8 patients who had RA. The mean time to fusion was 10 weeks and the investigators noted 100% arthrodesis rate with no complications. Dent and colleagues [45] reported on eight arthroscopic ankle fusions and also noted 100% fusion rate. Two of these patients had RA as a primary etiology. Jerosch and colleagues [55] reported on 26 patients (4 who had RA) who were treated with arthroscopic ankle arthrodesis and noted bony fusion in 85%. These series indicate that in selected patients, arthroscopic ankle arthrodesis may provide more reliable fusion with fewer complications than a standard open technique.

External fixation

The use of external fixation in ankle arthrodesis has some theoretic advantages over internal fixation, including the ability to adjust the final position and add compression in the postoperative period. A final fusion without retained internal hardware also has distinct advantages in this immunosuppressed population who has significantly increased rates of superficial, deep, and late infections. Some types of external fixators allow the patient to fully weight-bear in the immediate postoperative period, which is distinctly advantageous in patients who have contralateral pathology and upper extremity pathology. The primary disadvantages are the same as with internal fixation. Pin site infections can occur and cut out of half-pins and tensioned wires may be complications caused by osteoporosis and immunosuppression. Reported results for arthrodesis with external compression devices are similar for open procedures. Cracchiolo and colleagues [41] reviewed 32 patients who had ankle arthrodesis secondary to RA. Seventeen fusions were done by external fixation and 12 had fusion by internal fixation with screws. Four of 18 developed nonunion in the external fixation group, and all nonunions were associated with infection. Other complications included malunion and neurapraxia. The internal fixation group had a similar nonunion rate, with 3 of 12 ankles developing nonunion, but with only 1 developing infection. Two developed malunion in valgus. Dereymaeker and colleagues [33] reported on 14 ankle fusions done in 13 patients who had RA using an external fixation device or cannulated screws. A 31% nonunion rate was reported; however, the investigators reported significant improvement in union with the use of a fibular strut graft. Smith and Wood reviewed 11 patients who had severe RA of the ankle joint undergoing fusion with a Charnley compression device for external fixation [56]. All patients achieved bony union, although 4 of 11 had pin tract infections; this was the most frequent complication. Felix and Kitaoka reviewed ankle fusions in patients who had RA using internal and external fixation and reported on 12 ankle fusions and 14 tibiotalocalcaneal fusions [57]. Union rate was high with internal and external fixation, and the investigators noted a 96% arthrodesis rate.

Fibular strut and sliding bone graft

The use of a fibular strut graft has been reported by several investigators to improve stability and fusion rates. As noted, Dereymaeker and colleagues [33] reported that the use of a fibular strut improved fusion rates using internal and external fixation. Maenpaa and colleagues [58] reviewed 130 ankle fusions in patients who had RA using staples and a fibular buttress graft. Ninety-two percent of patients fused primarily. These investigators noted malalignment as a primary problem in these patients, and when critically assessed, believed that attempting to accomplish too much hindfoot correction through the ankle joint was a significant reason for failure. Use of a vascularized fibular strut graft to achieve ankle arthrodesis in revision and salvage cases has also been described with success [59]. Other investigators have reported on the use of a sliding tibial autograft to improve arthrodesis and to avoid the use of autogenous iliac crest grafts [19,60].

Other techniques

Other techniques have been described for fusion with varying results. Carrier reported a high success rate in 5 of 5 patients who had RA, successfully achieving fusion using only vertically aligned Steinman pins for fixation [61]. Dowel type arthrodesis was attempted in nine cases by Belt and colleagues [62] and was noted to have a high complication rate and a 32% nonunion rate. These investigators believed the results of this technique in patients who had RA were unacceptable. Fujimori and colleagues [27] reported on a nail specially designed for ankle fusion in 15 patients who had RA. Immediate weightbearing was allowed in most patients. Other investigators have reported results with fixation by blade plate with good success, although these series had arthritis from multiple etiologies [29,63]. All patients obtained a stable arthrodesis, and complications were self-limited and minor. Lauge-Pederson has advocated fusion through percutaneous fixation alone without joint preparation for patients to minimize complications; this is under investigation [64].

The author's preferred techniques

Isolated ankle arthrodesis is an uncommon procedure in patients who have RA for various reasons. It is unusual for pathology to be confined to the ankle joint. The ideal indications are intractable pain caused by loss of cartilage with minimal deformity. These cases can usually be managed with arthroscopic or "mini-open" joint preparation as described by Myerson and colleagues [48,65–67]. Any deformity or apparent bone loss on radiographs is treated with an open procedure with a transfibular approach and lateral fibular onlay graft. Varus deformity of more than 10° or valgus of more than 15° may need to be extended to a tibiotalocalcaneal fusion, which is typically done with an intramedullary hindfoot fusion rod or lateral blade plate. Arthritis or deformity at the level of the transverse tarsal joint may require a pan-talar arthrodesis.

The arthroscopic technique is performed through the anterolateral and anteromedial portals and a third posterolateral portal to facilitate adequate fluid flow. Mechanical distraction is helpful and the author uses an external fixator for this. Ankle joint distraction of 1.0 to 1.5 cm is typically tolerated and affords excellent visualization. Any remaining cartilage is removed with arthroscopic shavers, burs, and curettes, taking care to preserve the overall shape of the ankle. Thermal necrosis from the motorized bur has been a concern and may lead to nonunion. This is typically more of a concern in osteoarthritis than in RA because of the osteoporosis present with the latter. A low-pressure, high-flow arthroscopic fluid system is facilitated by a separate outflow cannula and helps minimize tissue temperature and keep the field of view clear of debris. The cartilage and subchondral bone are denuded to healthy-appearing cancellous surfaces. Osteophytes may be resected with a bur to facilitate proper positioning; in particular, anterior osteophytes may predispose to a final fusion in plantar flexion and should be removed before fixation. A C-arm fluoroscopy and an arthroscopic guide facilitate the placement of screws for fixation (Fig. 2).

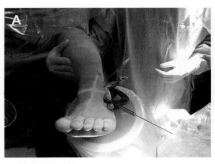 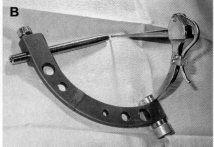

Fig. 2. Set up for arthroscopic ankle arthrodesis. (*A*) C-arm and arthroscopic guide for wire placement are useful in screw placement. (*B*) Micro-vector drill guide for small joint arthroscopy (*Courtesy of* Smith & Nephew, Memphis, TN; with permission).

The mini-arthrotomy technique is performed through two small incisions (2–3 cm) at the arthroscopy portal sites and allows for joint preparation with handheld tools, such as chisels, osteotomes, and curettes. The joint is distracted with small laminar spreaders. The risk for thermal injury with this technique is eliminated, excision of osteophytes is easier, and the author finds the positioning of the hardware and final arthrodesis position is faster. Fixation is by internal fixation with three compression screws: one applied from the lateral malleolus to the posteromedial talus, one from the medial malleolus to the lateral talar body, and a third from the posterior malleolus through the body into the talar neck and head (the "home run" screw) (Fig. 3). The addition of autogenous bone graft is not necessary if the joint contours are maintained and the arthrodesis fits together well with good apposition. If graft is needed, the author has seen no difference in the use of demineralized allogenic bone matrix over autograft.

For cases in which significant deformity is present, the author finds an open approach is best, because it allows balanced bone resection to achieve adequate alignment (Fig. 4). The patient is positioned semi-laterally on a bean bag and a straight incision is made over the fibula. The fibula is left in anatomic continuity with its posterior soft-tissue attachments so that it can be used as a vascularized corticocancellous graft. The distal 8 cm of fibula is freed from its distal ligamentous attachments circumferentially, including the lateral ankle ligaments, anterior and posterior tibiofibular ligaments, and interosseous membrane, taking care to leave the periosteum intact. The conjoined retinacular attachments of the inferior peroneal retinaculum and Achilles retinaculum are left intact to preserve blood supply to the fibula. The fibula is osteotomized 4 or 5 cm proximal to the joint surface, and the medial third, including the fibular articular surface, is resected with an oscillating saw. The remaining fibula is retracted posteriorly with the soft-tissue envelope and a subperiosteal dissection is then performed anteriorly and posteriorly about the distal tibia, taking

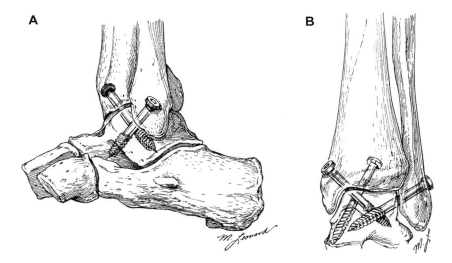

Fig. 3. Screw placement for ankle arthrodesis. (*A*) Two-screw technique. (*B*) Three-screw tech-nique with "home run" screw from posterior malleolus into talar neck and head. (*Reprinted from* Quill GE. An approach to the management of ankle arthritis. In: Myerson MS, editor. Foot and ankle disorders. Philadelphia: WB Saunders Co.; 2000. p. 1071, Figs. 44–17; with permission.)

care to release the entire joint capsule from the tibia. This affords an excel-lent exposure of the entire joint through a single plane dissection. The joint is spread with a laminar spreader, and the articular surfaces and osteophytes are resected using chisels and curettes. If varus deformity is present, bone may be resected laterally to correct up to 10°. If valgus deformity is present, medial bone can be resected, although if more than 10° correction is required, it may be necessary to osteotomize or remove the medial malleolus to prevent gapping as the talus is compressed to the tibia. Fixation is typi-cally with two or three screws. During closure, the incisura fibularis is re-sected to allow close compression of the fibular strut graft, and the lateral tibial cortex is feathered with a chisel to promote a fusion of the tibio-fibular joint. The fibular onlay graft is then secured to the lateral arthrodesis with 4-mm compression screws. Postoperatively patients are kept non-weightbearing in a short leg cast until radiographic union is achieved, typically at 8 to 12 weeks.

The author reserves the use of external fixation for specific cases in which internal fixation is contraindicated. These include patients who have a recent history of joint infection, open wounds, or a compromised soft-tissue enve-lope in which wound healing problems are anticipated. The most frequent application of this technique in the author's experience is for salvage of infected or failed ankle replacement or following severe ankle trauma, such as pilon fracture with soft-tissue compromise (Fig. 5). Bone quality and pin site infection can be problematic, and the surgeon should apply adequate fixation proximally and distally. Typically the author uses two tibial rings with crossed wires and one or two half pins. The hindfoot is fixed with crossed tensioned olive wires in the calcaneus, and if possible, a half pin or wires in the talar neck. The advantage of this technique is that immediate

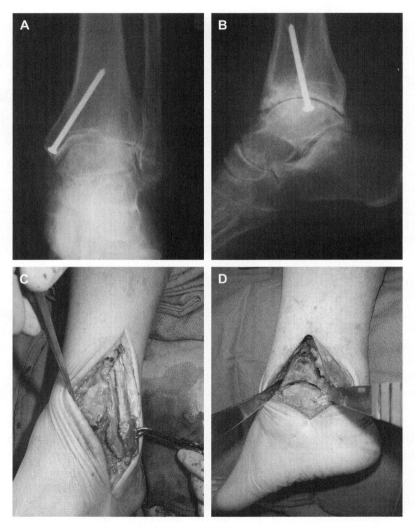

Fig. 4. Open arthrodesis with fibular onlay graft. (*A*, *B*) Preoperative films in a 65-year-old woman who had rheumatic disease and post-traumatic arthritis. (*C*) Lateral approach. The fibula has been released distally and split longitudinally. This allows it to be hinged posteriorly on the retinacular attachments. (*D*) Articular surfaces are resected with handheld tools, preserving joint architecture as much as possible. (*E*) Ankle joint exposure is facilitated by use of a laminar spreader. (*F*) The fibular graft is secured with compression screws laterally. (*G*, *H*) Postoperative films showing bony fusion and incorporation of the fibular graft.

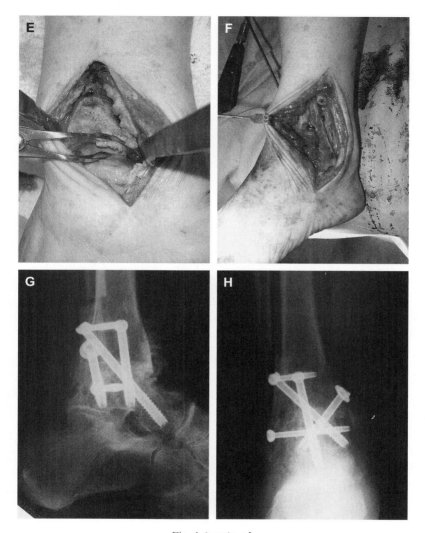

Fig. 4 (*continued*)

weightbearing can be allowed, although a sole for walking may need to be constructed to allow for clearance of the fixation devices.

Tibiotalocalcaneal arthrodesis is typically reserved for patients who have arthritic involvement of the subtalar joint [68]. For severe deformity with significant bone loss in which adequate fixation or stability may not be achieved through standard ankle fusion techniques, the author sometimes extends the arthrodesis of the ankle to include the subtalar joint. This simplifies alignment, and incorporation of the calcaneus dramatically improves

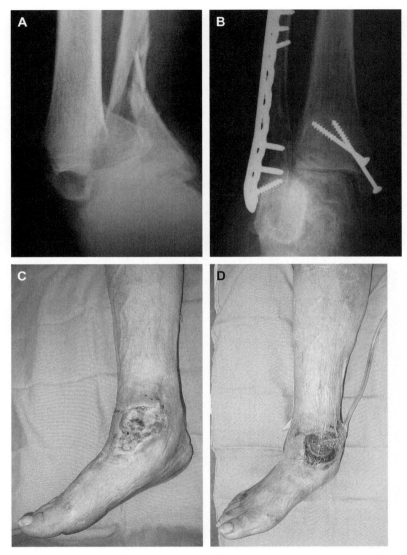

Fig. 5. Bimalleolar ankle fracture in a 58-year-old woman who had rheumatoid disease. (*A*, *B*) Preoperative and immediate postoperative radiographs. (*C*) Postsurgical photo showing loss of skin and exposed hardware. (*D*) Staged reconstruction involves initial debridement and application of a Wound Vac system (Kinetics Concepts Inc., San Antonio, TX). (*E*, *F*) Surgical arthrodesis is performed with Ilizarov ringed external fixator (Smith & Nephew, Memphis, TN) and organism-specific antibiotics. Wounds closed with split thickness graft over granulation tissue at 8 weeks. (*G*) Final radiographs showing fusion.

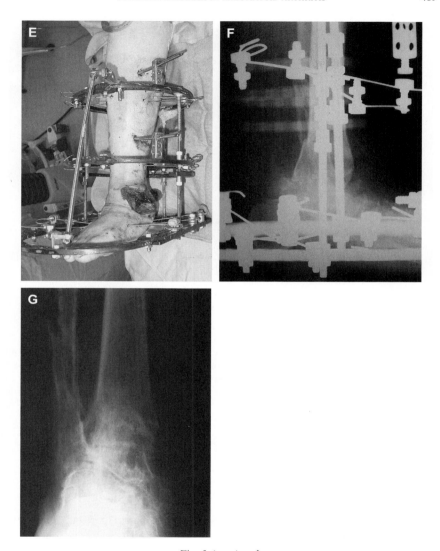

Fig. 5 (*continued*)

fixation and fusion rates [26,28]. The author has done this for failed ankle replacement, avascular necrosis of the talus, and severe deformity following trauma with good results (Fig. 6). In these cases, the surgeon must balance the potential morbidity associated with loss of subtalar motion versus the risk for failure of the primary procedure and the potential for further surgery and its associated risks and recovery.

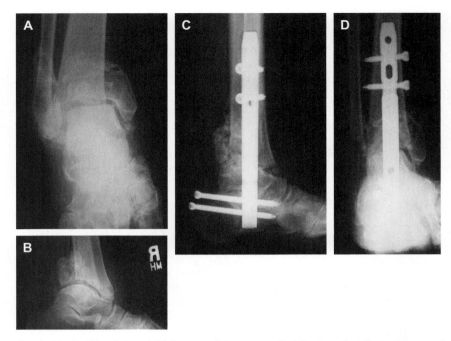

Fig. 6. (*A, B*) Pilon injury initially treated in cast resulted in posterior displacement and shortening. Vascular insufficiency precluded surgery at the time. Six weeks postinjury, patient is referred for amputation. (*C*) Endovascular procedure performed to improve blood flow to extremity. (*D, E*) Fusion with intramedullary rod done as salvage with radiographic fusion evident at 10 weeks.

Management of complications

Patients who have RA are at increased risk for complications, and management of those complications can be challenging. Soft-tissue complications are most typically related to wound dehiscence or necrosis of the soft-tissue envelope. Decreasing antirheumatic medications before surgery and for a period of time following surgery may decrease problems with wound healing and improve the chances of a poorly healing wound to resolve. Local wound care is advocated, but if no progress is made, adjuvant therapy, including specialized dressings, topical medications and gels, therapeutic modalities, and hyperbaric oxygen, should be considered [69]. Full thickness necrosis to hardware or bone invariably requires revision surgery. Debridement of necrotic tissue with rotational or free soft-tissue coverage is often necessary. Unfortunately the compromised host makes the likelihood of success for large soft-tissue loss tenuous and amputation can be the result.

   Nonunion is also a common complication. Revision surgery must address
the underlying cause of the failure. The author routinely works up immuno-
compromised patients presenting with nonunion for infection, because they
may not present with the normal signs and symptoms associated with
osteomyelitis. If infection is present, it must be eradicated before achieving
a successful fusion. In the author's experience, this is accomplished by debridement and fusion with a ringed external fixator. Compression can be

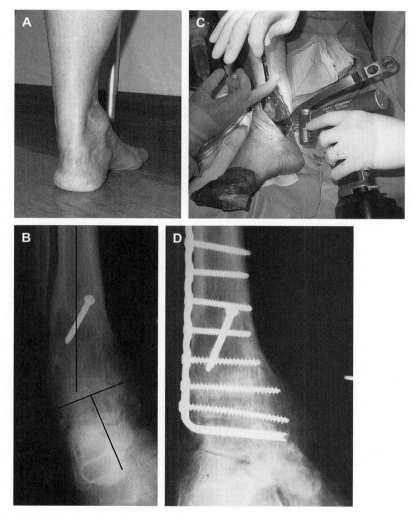

Fig. 7. Malunion in solid arthrodesis. Patient presented 7 years after successful arthrodesis with
painful malunion. Initial films seemed to have adequate alignment. (*A*) Clinical presentation
and radiographs showing varus malunion. (*B*) Radiographs showing varus malunion. (*C*)
Lateral closing wedge osteotomy is done. (*D*) Final alignment with blade plate.

added during the recovery period, and organism-specific antibiotics are continued until bony union becomes apparent, typically at 8 to 12 weeks.

In a sterile nonunion, if alignment is good and the fixation is stable 4 or 5 months following surgery, arthrodesis may be achieved by bone grafting the site with iliac crest graft. If the fixation is loose or alignment is deteriorating, formal revision and bone grafting is recommended with re-exposure of the arthrodesis site and revision of the fixation. Talar fixation can be problematic if the screws have pulled out. Better fixation can be achieved with a posteriorly applied blade plate, although consideration should be given at this point to extending the fusion to include the subtalar joint.

Many investigators note malunion as a common problem [58,70]. The author has seen patients who initially healed in good position subside into varus or valgus because of osteoporosis in the year following their initial surgery. If stable fusion has been achieved and the apex of the deformity is at the tibiotalar fusion site, the alignment can be corrected by supramalleolar osteotomy (Fig. 7).

Summary

Ankle arthrodesis remains a valuable tool in the management of patients who have RA. The primary indications include pain, deformity, and radiographic changes that preclude the success of other joint-sparing procedures. Although total ankle arthroplasty has gained some popularity for the treatment of ankle arthritis, its use in patients who have RA continues to be problematic for various reasons. Achieving a successful arthrodesis can be difficult but does provide lasting pain relief and deformity correction for these patients when successful.

References

[1] Jaakkola JI, Mann RA. A review of rheumatoid arthritis affecting the foot and ankle. Foot Ankle Int 2004;25:866–74.

[2] Rana NA. Juvenile rheumatoid arthritis of the foot. Foot Ankle 1982;3:2–11.

[3] Miehlke W, Gschwend N, Rippstein P, et al. Compression arthrodesis of the rheumatoid ankle and hindfoot. Clin Orthop Relat Res 1997;75–86.

[4] Vainio K. The rheumatoid foot: a clinical study with pathologic and rheumatologic comments. Ann Chir Gynaecol Suppl 1956;45:1.

[5] Abdo RV, Iorio LJ. Rheumatoid arthritis of the foot and ankle. J Am Acad Orthop Surg 1994;2:326–32.

[6] Thompson FM, Mann RA. Chapter 14: arthritides. In: Mann RA, Coughlin MJ, editors. Surgery of the foot and ankle. 6th edition. St. Louis (MO): Mosby; 1993. p. 615–71.

[7] Nassar J, Cracchiolo A 3rd. Complications in surgery of the foot and ankle in patients with rheumatoid arthritis. Clin Orthop Relat Res 2001;140–52.

[8] Galvin EM, O' Donnell D, Leonard IE. Rheumatoid arthritis: a significant but often underestimated risk factor for perioperative cardiac morbidity. Anesthesiology 2005;103:910–1.

[9] Bely M, Apathy A, Beke-Martos E. Cardiac changes in rheumatoid arthritis. Acta Morphol Hung 1992;40:149–86.

[10] Kramer PH, Imboden JB Jr, Waldman FM, et al. Severe aortic insufficiency in juvenile chronic arthritis. Am J Med 1983;74:1088–91.

[11] Mikulowski P, Wollheim FA, Rotmil P, et al. Sudden death in rheumatoid arthritis with atlanto-axial dislocation. Acta Med Scand 1975;198:445–51.

[12] Kauppi MJ, Barcelos A, da Silva JA. Cervical complications of rheumatoid arthritis. Ann Rheum Dis 2005;64:355–8.

[13] Kwek TK, Lew TW, Thoo FL. The role of preoperative cervical spine X-rays in rheumatoid arthritis. Anaesth Intensive Care 1998;26:636–41.

[14] Howe CR, Gardner GC, Kadel NJ. Perioperative medication management for the patient with rheumatoid arthritis. J Am Acad Orthop Surg 2006;14:544–51.

[15] McCauliffe DP, Sontheimer RD. Dermatologic manifestations of rheumatic disorders. Prim Care 1993;20:925–41.

[16] Henke PK, Sukheepod P, Proctor MC, et al. Clinical relevance of peripheral vascular occlusive disease in patients with rheumatoid arthritis and systemic lupus erythematosus. J Vasc Surg 2003;38:111–5.

[17] del Rincon I, Haas RW, Pogosian S, et al. Lower limb arterial incompressibility and obstruction in rheumatoid arthritis. Ann Rheum Dis 2005;64:425–32.

[18] Groth HE, Fitch HF. Salvage procedures for complications of total ankle arthroplasty. Clin Orthop Relat Res 1987;244–50.

[19] Iwata H, Yasuhara N, Kawashima K, et al. Arthrodesis of the ankle joint with rheumatoid arthritis: experience with the transfibular approach. Clin Orthop Relat Res 1980;189–93.

[20] Bogoch ER, Moran EL. Bone abnormalities in the surgical treatment of patients with rheumatoid arthritis. Clin Orthop Relat Res 1999;8–21.

[21] Deodhar AA, Woolf AD. Bone mass measurement and bone metabolism in rheumatoid arthritis: a review. Br J Rheumatol 1996;35:309–22.

[22] Benvenuti S, Brandi ML. Corticosteroid-induced osteoporosis: pathogenesis and prevention. Clin Exp Rheumatol 2000;18:S64–6.

[23] Dequeker J, Maenaut K, Verwilghen J, et al. Osteoporosis in rheumatoid arthritis. Clin Exp Rheumatol 1995;13(Suppl 12):S21–6.

[24] Urquhart MW, Mont MA, Michelson JD, et al. Osteonecrosis of the talus: treatment by hindfoot fusion. Foot Ankle Int 1996;17:275–82.

[25] Anderson T, Maxander P, Rydholm U, et al. Ankle arthrodesis by compression screws in rheumatoid arthritis: primary nonunion in 9/35 patients. Acta Orthop 2005;76: 884–90.

[26] Anderson T, Linder L, Rydholm U, et al. Tibio-talocalcaneal arthrodesis as a primary procedure using a retrograde intramedullary nail: a retrospective study of 26 patients with rheumatoid arthritis. Acta Orthop 2005;76:580–7.

[27] Fujimori J, Yoshino S, Koiwa M, et al. Ankle arthrodesis in rheumatoid arthritis using an intramedullary nail with fins. Foot Ankle Int 1999;20:485–90.

[28] Moore TJ, Prince R, Pochatko D, et al. Retrograde intramedullary nailing for ankle arthrodesis. Foot Ankle Int 1995;16:433–6.

[29] Sowa DT, Krackow KA. Ankle fusion: a new technique of internal fixation using a compression blade plate. Foot Ankle 1989;9:232–40.

[30] Ahmad J, Pour AI, Raikin SM. The use of a modified locking plate to achieve tibiotalocalcaneal arthrodesis. Presented at the American Orthopaedic Foot And Ankle Society summer meeting. La Jolla, CA, July 14–16, 2006.

[31] Hertel R, Jost B. Basic principles and techniques in fixation of osteoporotic bone. New York: Thieme; 2002. p. 108–15.

[32] Braly WG, Baker JK, Tullos HS. Arthrodesis of the ankle with lateral plating. Foot Ankle Int 1994;15:649–53.

[33] Dereymaeker GP, Van Eygen P, Driesen R, et al. Tibiotalar arthrodesis in the rheumatoid foot. Clin Orthop Relat Res 1998;43–7.

[34] Thordarson DB, Markolf KL, Cracchiolo A 3rd. Arthrodesis of the ankle with cancellous-bone screws and fibular strut graft. Biomechanical analysis. J Bone Joint Surg Am 1990;72: 1359–63.

[35] Moran CG, Pinder IM, Smith SR. Ankle arthrodesis in rheumatoid arthritis. 30 cases followed for 5 years. Acta Orthop Scand 1991;62:538–43.

[36] Chen YJ, Huang TJ, Shih HN, et al. Ankle arthrodesis with cross screw fixation. Good results in 36/40 cases followed 3–7 years. Acta Orthop Scand 1996;67:473–8.

[37] Kennedy JG, Harty JA, Casey K, et al. Outcome after single technique ankle arthrodesis in patients with rheumatoid arthritis. Clin Orthop Relat Res 2003;131–8.

[38] Maurer RC, Cimino WR, Cox CV, et al. Transarticular cross-screw fixation. A technique of ankle arthrodesis. Clin Orthop Relat Res 1991;56–64.

[39] Kennedy JG, Hodgkins CW, Brodsky A, et al. Outcomes after standardized screw fixation technique of ankle arthrodesis. Clin Orthop Relat Res 2006;447:112–8.

[40] Holt ES, Hansen ST, Mayo KA, et al. Ankle arthrodesis using internal screw fixation. Clin Orthop Relat Res 1991;21–8.

[41] Cracchiolo A 3rd, Cimino WR, Lian G. Arthrodesis of the ankle in patients who have rheumatoid arthritis. J Bone Joint Surg Am 1992;74:903–9.

[42] Partio EK, Hirvensalo E, Partio E, et al. Talocrural arthrodesis with absorbable screws, 12 cases followed for 1 year. Acta Orthop Scand 1992;63:170–2.

[43] Corso SJ, Zimmer TJ. Technique and clinical evaluation of arthroscopic ankle arthrodesis. Arthroscopy 1995;11:585–90.

[44] Cameron SE, Ullrich P. Arthroscopic arthrodesis of the ankle joint. Arthroscopy 2000;16: 21–6.

[45] Dent CM, Patil M, Fairclough JA. Arthroscopic ankle arthrodesis. J Bone Joint Surg Br 1993;75:830–2.

[46] Jay RM. A new concept of ankle arthrodesis via arthroscopic technique. Clin Podiatr Med Surg 2000;17:147–57, vii.

[47] Raikin SM. Arthrodesis of the ankle: arthroscopic, mini-open, and open techniques. Foot Ankle Clin 2003;8:347–59.

[48] Myerson MS, Quill G. Ankle arthrodesis. A comparison of an arthroscopic and an open method of treatment. Clin Orthop Relat Res 1991;84–95.

[49] O'Brien TS, Hart TS, Shereff MJ, et al. Open versus arthroscopic ankle arthrodesis: a comparative study. Foot Ankle Int 1999;20:368–74.

[50] Winson IG, Robinson DE, Allen PE. Arthroscopic ankle arthrodesis. J Bone Joint Surg Br 2005;87:343–7.

[51] Tasto JP, Frey C, Laimans P, et al. Arthroscopic ankle arthrodesis. Instr Course Lect 2000; 49:259–80.

[52] De Vriese L, Dereymaeker G, Fabry G. Arthroscopic ankle arthrodesis. Preliminary report. Acta Orthop Belg 1994;60:389–92.

[53] Stone JW. Arthroscopic ankle arthrodesis. Foot Ankle Clin 2006;11:361–8, vi–vii.

[54] Turan I, Wredmark T, Fellander-Tsai L. Arthroscopic ankle arthrodesis in rheumatoid arthritis. Clin Orthop Relat Res 1995;110–4.

[55] Jerosch J, Steinbeck J, Schroder M, et al. Arthroscopically assisted arthrodesis of the ankle joint. Arch Orthop Trauma Surg 1996;115:182–9.

[56] Smith EJ, Wood PL. Ankle arthrodesis in the rheumatoid patient. Foot Ankle 1990;10: 252–6.

[57] Felix NA, Kitaoka HB. Ankle arthrodesis in patients with rheumatoid arthritis. Clin Orthop Relat Res 1998;58–64.

[58] Maenpaa H, Lehto MU, Belt EA. Why do ankle arthrodeses fail in patients with rheumatic disease? Foot Ankle Int 2001;22:403–8.

[59] Yajima H, Kobata Y, Tomita Y, et al. Ankle and pantalar arthrodeses using vascularized fibular grafts. Foot Ankle Int 2004;25:3–7.

[60] Patterson BM, Inglis AE, Moeckel BH. Anterior sliding graft for tibiotalar arthrodesis. Foot Ankle Int 1997;18:330–4.
[61] Carrier DA, Harris CM. Ankle arthrodesis with vertical Steinmann's pins in rheumatoid arthritis. Clin Orthop Relat Res 1991;10–4.
[62] Belt EA, Maenpaa H, Lehto MU. Outcome of ankle arthrodesis performed by dowel technique in patients with rheumatic disease. Foot Ankle Int 2001;22:666–9.
[63] Weltmer JB Jr, Choi SH, Shenoy A, et al. Wolf blade plate ankle arthrodesis. Clin Orthop Relat Res 1991;107–11.
[64] Lauge-Pedersen H. Percutaneous arthrodesis. Acta Orthop Scand Suppl 2003;74(Suppl I): 1–30.
[65] Glick JM, Morgan CD, Myerson MS, et al. Ankle arthrodesis using an arthroscopic method: long-term follow-up of 34 cases. Arthroscopy 1996;12:428–34.
[66] Paremain GD, Miller SD, Myerson MS. Ankle arthrodesis: results after the miniarthrotomy technique. Foot Ankle Int 1996;17:247–52.
[67] Miller SD, Paremain GP, Myerson MS. The miniarthrotomy technique of ankle arthrodesis: a cadaver study of operative vascular compromise and early clinical results. Orthopedics 1996;19:425–30.
[68] Chou LB, Mann RA, Yaszay B, et al. Tibiotalocalcaneal arthrodesis. Foot Ankle Int 2000; 21:804–8.
[69] Hess CL, Howard MA, Attinger CE. A review of mechanical adjuncts in wound healing: hydrotherapy, ultrasound, negative pressure therapy, hyperbaric oxygen, and electrostimulation. Ann Plast Surg 2003;51:210–8.
[70] Dennis DA, Clayton ML, Wong DA, et al. Internal fixation compression arthrodesis of the ankle. Clin Orthop Relat Res 1990;212–20.

**ELSEVIER
SAUNDERS**

Foot Ankle Clin N Am
12 (2007) 497–508

**FOOT AND
ANKLE CLINICS**

Total Ankle Replacement
for Rheumatoid Ankle Arthritis

Peter L.R. Wood, MB, BS, FRCS*,
Louise A. Crawford, MB, ChB, MRSC (Ed),
Rajeev Suneja, MS(Orth), MSC(Tr), FRCS(Tr&Orth),
Ann Kenyon, BSc, MA

Wrightington Hospital Wigan, Hall Lane, Appley Bridge, Wigan, WN6 9EP, UK

Polyarticular rheumatoid arthritis affects the ankle in 15% to 52% of patients but rarely arises in the early course of the disease [1–3]. The patient has typically undergone prolonged medical treatment and may have osteoporosis, fragile skin, and a poor soft-tissue envelope around the ankle. Both ankles are often affected and arthritic change is also seen in the upper and lower limbs, and these have often been treated by arthroplasty before severe ankle symptoms develop [4]. In the rheumatoid population as a whole, many ankles do remain in neutral alignment, but it is the combination of deformity and joint destruction that produces the most severe symptoms. Valgus deformity frequently develops and may be associated with rupture of the deltoid ligament and stress fracture of the fibula. In a review of 150 patients attending a special hospital for patients who have rheumatoid diseases, Kirkup [1] found that valgus deformity had developed three times more frequently than varus. Valgus deformity was seen in 50% of the authors' patients who have rheumatoid arthritis who required surgical treatment by either fusion or replacement. Varus deformity on the other hand was present in only 20%.

It is usual for the rheumatoid condition to damage the ankle joints and those of the hindfoot simultaneously. In the authors' practice, 90% of patients had obvious radiologic arthritic change in the hindfoot, 30% had spontaneous fusion of the subtalar joint, and 10% had undergone a previous surgical fusion. This has also been reported elsewhere in the literature [5,6].

---

* Corresponding author.
E-mail address: peter.wood@wwl.nhs.uk (P.L.R. Wood).

1083-7515/07/$ - see front matter © 2007 Elsevier Inc. All rights reserved.
doi:10.1016/j.fcl.2007.05.002

Preoperative workup

The preoperative work-up for patients undergoing total ankle joint replacement for rheumatoid arthritis must include a careful assessment of the systemic effects of the rheumatoid disease. Surgery, particularly joint replacement, should be avoided in the presence of vasculitis or severe neuropathy. Provided there is no major bone loss or stiffness, Bonnin [7] advises that replacement should be recommended to all patients who have rheumatoid arthritis for whom conservative treatment has failed. This view is not universally held, and arguably ankle fusion may be preferable for the patient who has rheumatoid arthritis with severe polyarthritis and systemic disease. In such cases coexisting problems restrict the scope for restoration of normal activity, and ankle fusion offers a way for these patients to regain the ability to walk indoors without pain. For these patients specifically, it is the authors' opinion that it is unjustified to carry out replacement, because the complications are more frequent and generally more difficult to resolve than those following fusion. Most patients are able to walk moderate distances outdoors once their ankle pain has been relieved. An ankle fusion, however, may make climbing steps and negotiating uneven surfaces difficult. Moreover there would be additional stresses on the joints of the hindfoot that have already been affected by the rheumatoid process, and these could soon become painful. In most instances, therefore, maintenance of movement at the ankle by way of a successful ankle joint replacement is highly beneficial.

Notwithstanding the desirability of performing a replacement, severe destruction of bone such as extensive bone cysts in the talus may preclude there being a successful durable result because of the lack of adequate bony support for the prosthesis. The most frequently encountered contraindication with respect to the anatomy of the joint itself is the presence of valgus or varus deformity. This has repeatedly been demonstrated as carrying a high risk for failure because of recurrent deformity and instability [4,6,8–10]. Weight-bearing radiographs are obligatory if the deformity is to be measured accurately [1]. Doets and colleagues [6] estimates the deformity by identifying the joint line on the anteroposterior (AP) radiograph and advises that replacement is contraindicated when the deformity is greater than 10°. The joint line is often ill defined as a result of bony erosion, and so the authors have used a method of measurement relying on the sidewalls of the talus, because they are usually well preserved and easily identified (Fig. 1). Measured in this way, the authors regard 20° or more as an absolute contraindication to ankle arthroplasty. Other surgeons may have a different cut-off point, but it is agreed that when the deltoid ligament is disrupted, ankle replacement is contraindicated [11].

The presence of coexisting severe arthritic change in the ankle and hindfoot is perhaps the most notable difference between rheumatoid and osteoarthritic patients. Assessment of the condition of the subtalar and midtarsal joints is

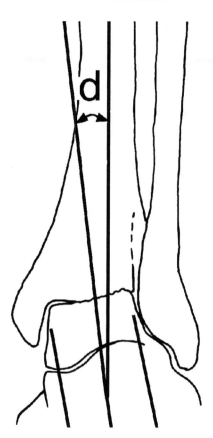

Fig. 1. Angle *d* measures the deformity. It is necessarily an estimate, because the arthritic process often distorts the outline of the talus. (*From* Wood PLR. Total ankle replacement: experience with the STAR ankle arthroplasty at Wrightington Hospital, UK. Foot Ankle Clin 2002;7(4):757; with permission.)

essential, because any deformity of the hindfoot profoundly influences the extent of treatment required. Clinical examination and standing AP radiographs may give sufficient information, but CT or MRI scans offer a more comprehensive picture. It is sometimes the case that pain is also arising from the talonavicular joint, and in 10% of cases the authors carry out an isolated fusion of that joint at the time of the replacement. The technique is straightforward and adds little to the postoperative morbidity. The incision is extended a short way distally, and the bone removed from the distal tibia is used as a graft. Internal fixation is with a staple. In the authors' practice, however, we have not fused the subtalar joint when it was anatomically well aligned even if the radiographs show arthritic change, and in almost every instance, patients have obtained an entirely satisfactory result. There is, however, no consensus view; Bonnin [7] believes that fusion of the hindfoot is necessary for most patients who have rheumatoid arthritis before ankle replacement, and others perform it in more than 25% of cases [12].

It is universally agreed, however, that ankle replacement demands that the heel is well aligned under the tibia. When the hindfoot is in severe planovalgus this must be corrected by hindfoot fusion. This can be done at the time of the replacement as a one-stage procedure [5,13], but it may be safer to stage the surgery and carry out the fusion 6 or 12 weeks before the ankle replacement [5–7,14]. The authors have done this on occasion, but it is often decided to perform a tibiotalocalcaneal fusion after discussion with the patient because of their general health problems and the wish to keep the number of operations to a minimum.

It is, however, generally considered that fusion is often a sensible option for a painful ankle that is also stiff; this is for two reasons. First, the range of motion improves only slightly after joint replacement [4,12,15,16], and second, replacement requires a more extensive surgical exposure than fusion, increasing the risk for wound breakdown. These factors, however, must be weighed against the fact that when the remainder of the foot is ankylosed, even 15° arc of motion is of value so long as it is centered on the neutral position.

In brief

Despite the caveats mentioned, there are many patients who have rheumatoid arthritis for whom replacement has clear and undeniable advantages over fusion. In the authors' practice the ratio of replacement to fusion is approximately 3:1. The ideal indication for rheumatoid ankle joint replacement is a moderately active rheumatoid patient who has a well-aligned ankle and heel. Some symptoms relating to the foot and ankle or knee will be apparently on the same or opposite leg. Fusing the ankle aggravates the impending arthritic problems in these joints and should therefore be avoided if possible. The pre- and postoperative radiographs of such a patient are shown in Fig. 2.

Recommendations regarding preoperative policy for antirheumatic medication

Methotrexate and corticosteroids are commonly used to control the inflammation of rheumatoid arthritis. Once control has been established, sudden cessation of their use may cause a flare-up of the disease, exacerbating pain and making postoperative rehabilitation more difficult. Early reports advise stopping methotrexate preoperatively in the belief that the immunosuppressive action of the drug increases the risk for infection [2]. Recent reports, however, have recommended continuing medication in the usual dosage [17,18]. In the authors' unit, long-term steroids and methotrexate are continued in their usual dosage throughout the perioperative period. Only for patients in whom there has been a recent increase in steroid

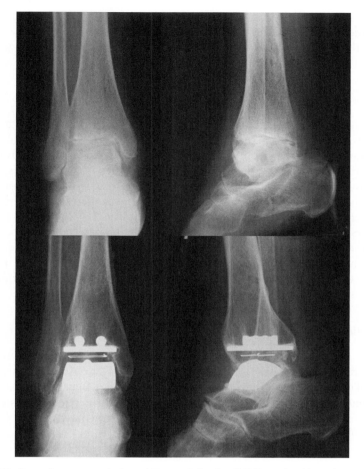

Fig. 2. Radiographs preoperatively and 7 years following STAR total ankle replacement with a good radiographic and clinical outcome.

requirement do the authors reconsider deferring surgery until medication requirements have stabilized.

By far the more current controversial debate regards the use of the newer disease modifying antirheumatic drugs (DMARDs), namely the anti-tumor necrosis factor (TNF) drugs. The authors follow the latest guidelines published by the British Society for Rheumatology [19]. These recommend that treatment with etanercept, adalimumab, and infliximab should be withheld before major surgical procedures for between 2 and 8 weeks depending on the half-life of the medication. Treatment may be restarted no sooner than 2 weeks postoperatively provided that there is no infection and the wound is healing satisfactorily. These guidelines will undoubtedly be modified as further studies are performed. For example, it has recently been reported that continued use of anti-TNF medication in the perioperative period did not increase the incidence of infection or wound complications in patients who had rheumatoid arthritis undergoing foot and ankle surgery [20].

Postoperative regime

It is generally advised that the ankle is immobilized in a cast for approximately 4 weeks postoperatively to rest the soft tissues. In the patient who has osteoarthritis, some surgeons recommend nonweightbearing. However, this is rarely an option for the patient who has rheumatoid arthritis, unless they use a wheelchair, because it would place too severe a strain on other joints, making them painful [12]. When this happens the symptoms may persist even when normal gait is once more established. The authors instruct patients to wear an Aircast (Vista, CA) below-knee walker for the first 2 weeks and weightbear as comfort permits. The walker boot is then worn while the patient is standing or walking for an additional 2 weeks. It is removed to wash the foot as necessary and for 10 minutes of dorsiflexion exercises twice a day. Sutures are removed between 3 and 4 weeks.

Wrightington Hospital results

Between 1993 and 2003 the authors performed 211 ankle joint replacements in patients who had rheumatoid arthritis. There were 171 Scandinavian Total Ankle Replacement (STAR) and 40 Beuchel-Pappas (BP) replacements. One hundred and nineteen of these formed part of a study reported in 2003 [4]. There were 158 replacements in women and 53 in men, and the average age was 58 years (range, 18–83 years). Thirty-six patients underwent staged bilateral replacements. Thirty-six patients died from unrelated causes during the follow-up period. Twenty ankles have failed; thus, the 8-year survivorship for the whole group is 88% (95% confidence interval [CI], 77%–99%). For those who had well-preserved preoperative alignment, survivorship at 8 years was 97% (80%–100%). There are only 34 patients who have a follow-up of longer than 8 years, and one of these failed at 9 years, giving a 10-year survivorship of 83% (CI, 60%–100%). There is no statistical difference in these results compared with patients who have osteoarthritis in the authors' institution.

The reasons for failure were early infection in two cases, late infection in one patient on anti-TNF medication, seven cases of aseptic loosening, eight cases of recurrent deformity associated with loosening, and two cases of broken polyethylene inserts in the STAR replacement.

Intraoperative malleolar fracture occurred in 9% of patients but healed without long-term consequences.

Wound healing problems occurred in 15% of patients in the early years. All of these patients' wounds eventually healed even though two cases took more than 6 months. The authors do not use skin grafts or flaps, because our previous experience with their use for patients who have rheumatoid arthritis has been poor.

The incidence of delayed wound healing has fallen dramatically over the years, undoubtedly because of improved surgical technique and tissue handling. The incidence is now 3% and healing has always been achieved by 2 months. Experience has also led to a similar reduction in the incidence of intraoperative malleolar fractures so that it is now a rare occurrence. The authors now resist any temptation to remove the fragment in one piece but rather extract it piecemeal starting from the lateral side, avoiding any tendency to lever against the medial malleolus. Late fracture occurring during the 6 months following surgery, however, remains a problem.

Eight-year survivorship

Various publications include only patients who have rheumatoid arthritis as the primary diagnosis and some others describe the outcomes for rheumatoid ankles separately from osteoarthritis. The 8-year survivorship with revision of components or conversion to fusion as an end-point has been in the range of 70%–93% [5,12,21]. It is notable that most of these studies involve series of less than 30 rheumatoid patients. There are two large studies. One from the Swedish Ankle Arthroplasty Register with 261 rheumatoid patients who had a 5-year survivorship of 82% (CI, 76%–98%) [8]. The other is from Doets and colleagues [6] who report an 8-year survivorship of 84% (CI, 73%–93%) in a series of 93 patients with rheumatoid arthritis. The survivorship, however, was much higher at 90% (CI, 82%–98%) in the subgroup whose alignment was well preserved. This figure is similar to the 93% reported in a study in which hindfoot malalignment of more than 10° was considered an absolute contraindication to ankle replacement [12]. Bonnin [7] reports a series of 32 ankles with a mean follow-up of 5 years in which the American Orthopedic Foot and Ankle Society (AOFAS) score for pain improved from 5 to 35 and for function from 24 to 43. These studies all relate to the three-component mobile bearing type of prosthesis. and the results are essentially the same as the authors'. A large study of the 132 Agility prosthesis in which 23% of patients had rheumatoid arthritis had a survivorship of 85% (CI, 71%–95%) at 10 years [22]. Unlike the designs of the 1970s when some reports suggested that the results were poorer in patients who had rheumatoid arthritis, recent studies with currently available prostheses have found no difference in outcome between patients who have rheumatoid arthritis and patients who have osteoarthritis [23–25].

Age of patient

Some investigators' reports have found poorer outcomes in younger patients [6,8,26], but others have not [27]. Assuming normal life expectancy, however, the younger patient requires a longer lasting result than an elderly patient if revision surgery is to be avoided. For patients who have rheumatoid arthritis the situation is different from those patients who have osteoarthritis, because activity is generally restricted by problems with other joints and life expectancy may be reduced. The authors' view on this is changing, however, in light of the improved life expectancy for patients who have rheumatoid arthritis because of advances in medical treatment [28].

Aseptic loosening, osteolysis and cortical support

The need to ensure that there is good cortical support of the tibial component has been stressed by several workers [6,12,16]. This is because a component that rests only on soft cancellous bone inevitably subsides. The level of the tibial resection is governed by the need to create sufficient space for the components and restore normal length and tension to the ligaments. Where the joint line is moved proximally in a valgus ankle by the depression on the tibial plafond, this resection may skirt the subarticular layer. In lax ankles the resection may similarly be right against the articular surface, but in the stiff tight ankle at least 3 mm of bone must be removed. This makes the exposed cancellous bone weak, and cortical support even amounting to leaving the component overhanging the bony margin anteriorly and posteriorly is vital.

Designs in which the talar component covers the full width of the bone and those that preserve the cortical sidewalls of the talus may be advantageous in that they give the maximum support possible. The Agility prosthesis has recently had its "footprint" extended with this in mind. The desire to have minimal bony resection and thereby preserve the strength of the subchondral bone is the driving force behind designs that require three faces to be cut on the talar surface, each with less than 2 mm resection. This adds complexity to the surgical procedure, but it is particularly important in rheumatoid ankles. It has been noticed that there may be some early talar and tibial subsidence that occurs in the first few postoperative months and then the components become stable [29].

A report of the TNK prosthesis, a ceramic on polyethylene fixed bearing design, is less encouraging, with tibial migration occurring in most and talar collapse in 9 of 21 ankles [30]. The addition of a hydroxyapatite coating to this prosthesis, however, has been reported to enhance its fixation to bone [31]. The STAR ankle as used in Europe has a calcium phosphate layer in addition to the titanium Porocoat.

There are no recommendations to use acrylic bone cement with any of the current prosthetic designs. This is because bone cement is only effective when a force can be applied perpendicular to the contact surface between implant and bone. For the ankle this would be along the weightbearing axis of the lower leg. To the best of the authors' knowledge, no way of carrying this out has yet been devised for the ankle, because any approach that enabled that to be done would be too destructive to the soft tissues.

Fractures

Intraoperative malleolar fracture is the most frequent complication to occur at the time of surgery. The medial malleolus is more at risk [6]. The osteopenia associated with rheumatoid arthritis makes the medial malleolus particularly vulnerable. It can be avulsed from the tibia by inadvertently over-distracting the ankle with bone spreaders while gaining exposure of the posterior part of the joint, or it may be snapped by levering against it while removing the bony fragments created by the distal tibial bone cut [32]. The incidence decreases with experience [33–35].

It has been suggested that this complication may be reduced by prophylactic pinning of the malleoli before beginning the saw cut, by careful attention to the excursion of the saw blade to avoid inadvertently cutting too far medially, and by careful distraction of the joint [12,32]. It is also important to avoid using components that are too large and encroach on the medial malleolus where it meets the tibial shaft. The risk for fracture may also be increased in patients who have rheumatoid arthritis who are on corticosteroids, and therefore in this particular group every care must be taken while preparing the tibial surface.

It is inconceivable that intraoperative fractures will be avoided altogether, and how they should be managed depends on the degree of displacement. Undisplaced fractures in which the soft-tissue sleeve is intact can be treated conservatively and rarely affect the long-term outcome [6,11]. In cases in which there is displacement, however, internal fixation is mandatory, because nonunion may occur, leading to instability of the joint. Some surgeons prefer to treat all fractures by tension band wiring or screw fixation [12].

The medial malleolus is weakened, because the resection removes the strong medial subchondral bone at the superomedial corner of the joint and this remodels gradually over the course of a few months. During this time a stress fracture may occur. It usually takes the form of an undisplaced crack running proximally and heals uneventfully with conservative treatment. If a fracture occurs many months after surgery, however, it may be caused by abnormal forces on the medial malleolus by malalignment of the components, and it then is an indication that the joint has failed. Salvage by fusion, or in favorable circumstances, revision, may be required.

Infection and wound dehiscence

Early deep infection is a risk with all joint replacements and perhaps particularly for patients who have rheumatoid arthritis with immunosuppression. The reported incidence of approximately 2% is similar to that for total knee replacement, and management is essentially along the same lines. Deep infection can occur later, and again the incidence is approximately 2%. The infection may settle without removal of components being necessary with surgical washout and antibiotics, but in approximately 1 in 4 cases conversion to an arthrodesis has been found necessary [5,6,12]. Delayed wound healing is a major problem for all surgeons but is universally reported as becoming less and less frequent as experience for each individual increases. Rotation flaps and skin grafts have sometimes been found necessary to achieve soft-tissue healing [12,35].

Summary

The benefits of replacement over fusion for the patient who has rheumatoid arthritis are undisputed. Recent reports have consistently shown that patient satisfaction is high and prosthetic survival is more than 90% at 5 years and in many instances more than 80% at 10 years. Preoperative assessment must of course ensure that bone and soft tissues are adequate to permit primary healing and to support the implant. Equally important, however, is assessment of the alignment of the ankle itself and the foot as a whole. Even moderate valgus or varus deformity at the ankle can significantly increase the likelihood of early failure and so does failing to surgically correct any valgus hindfoot deformity. One word of caution must be given, however, namely that patients who have rheumatoid arthritis often express a high level of satisfaction with their outcome even when objective measures such as radiographs are far from satisfactory [5,12,25,30]. This may come from a stoicism arising from their chronic disability or because they are generally lightly built and place low demands on the arthroplasty. The authors believe the future will show replacement to be a valuable option for the patient who has rheumatoid arthritis, but there are not yet a sufficient number of long-term studies to say that this is proven.

References

[1] Kirkup J. Rheumatoid arthritis and ankle surgery. Ann Rheum Dis 1990;49(Suppl 2): 837–44.
[2] Lachiewicz PF. Total ankle arthroplasty. Indications, techniques, and results. Orthop Rev 1994;23:315–20.
[3] Michelson J, Easley M, Wigley FM, et al. Foot and ankle problems in rheumatoid arthritis. Foot Ankle Int 1994;15(11):608–13.
[4] Wood PL, Deakin S. Total ankle replacement. The results in 200 ankles. J Bone Joint Surg Br 2003;85(3):334–41.
[5] Su EP, Kahn B, Figgie MP. Total ankle replacement in patients with rheumatoid arthritis. Clin Orthop Relat Res 2004;424:32–8.
[6] Doets HC, Brand R, Nelissen RG. Total ankle arthroplasty in inflammatory joint disease with use of two mobile-bearing designs. J Bone Joint Surg Am 2006;88(6): 1272–84.

[7] Bonnin M, Bouysset M, Tebib J, et al. Total ankle replacement in rheumatoid arthritis: treatment strategy. In: Bouysset M, Tourné Y, Tillmann K, editors. Foot and ankle in rheumatoid arthritis. Paris: Springer-Verlag; 2006. p. 206–19.

[8] Henricson A, Skoog A, Carlsson A. The Swedish ankle arthroplasty register: an analysis of 531 cases performed 1993-2005. Acta Orthop, in press.

[9] Henricson A, Agren P. Secondary surgery after total ankle replacement. The influence of preoperative hindfoot alignment. Foot Ankle Surgery 2007;13:41–4.

[10] Haskell A, Mann R. Ankle arthroplasty with preoperative coronal plane deformity. Clin Orthop Relat Res 2004;424:98–103.

[11] Greisberg J, Hansen S. Ankle replacement: management of associated deformities. Foot Ankle Clin 2002;7:721–36.

[12] San Giovanni TP, Keblish DJ, Thomas WH, et al. Eight-year results of a minimally constrained total ankle arthroplasty. Foot Ankle Int 2006;27(6):418–26.

[13] Hintermann B. Total ankle arthroplasty. Wien: Springer-Verlag; 2005. p. 93.

[14] Valtin B, Leemrijse T. Hindfoot surgery for rheumatoid arthritis. In: Bouysset M, Tourné Y, Tillmann K, editors. Foot and ankle in rheumatoid arthritis. Paris: Springer-Verlag; 2006. p. 149–67.

[15] Coetzee JC, Castro MD. Accurate measurement of ankle range of motion after total ankle arthroplasty. Clin Orthop Relat Res 2004;424:27–31.

[16] Anderson T, Montgomery F, Carlsson A. Uncemented STAR total ankle prostheses. Three- to eight-year follow-up of fifty-one consecutive ankles. J Bone Joint Surg Am 2003;85(7): 1321–9.

[17] Grennan DM, Gray J, Loudon J, et al. Methotrexate and early postoperative complications in patients with rheumatoid arthritis undergoing elective orthopaedic surgery. Ann Rheum Dis 2002;61(1):86–7.

[18] Jain A, Witbreuk M, Ball C, et al. Influence of steroids and methotrexate on wound complications after elective rheumatoid hand and wrist surgery. J Hand Surg [Am] 2002;27(3): 449–55.

[19] Ledingham J, Deighton C, British Society for Rheumatology Standards, Guidelines and Audit Working Group (SGAWG). Update on the British Society for Rheumatology guidelines for prescribing TNFα blockers in adults with rheumatoid arthritis (update of previous guidelines of April 2001). Rheumatology 2005;44:157–63.

[20] Bibbo C, Goldberg JW. Infectious and healing complications after elective orthopaedic foot and ankle surgery during tumor necrosis factor-alpha inhibition therapy. Foot Ankle Int 2004;25(5):331–5.

[21] Buechel FF Sr, Buechel FF Jr, Pappas MJ. Twenty-year evaluation of cementless mobile-bearing total ankle replacements. Clin Orthop Relat Res 2004;(424):19–26.

[22] Knecht SI, Estin M, Callaghan JJ, et al. The agility total ankle arthroplasty. Seven- to sixteen-year follow-up. J Bone Joint Surg Am 2004;86(6):1161–71.

[23] Stengel D, Bauwens K, Ekkernkamp A, et al. Efficacy of total ankle replacement with meniscal-bearing devices: a systematic review and meta-analysis. Arch Orthop Trauma Surg 2005;125(2):109–19 [Epub Feb 3, 2005].

[24] Kopp FJ, Patel MM, Deland JT, et al. Total ankle arthroplasty with the agility prosthesis: clinical and radiographic evaluation. Foot Ankle Int 2006;27(2):97–103.

[25] Kofoed H, Sorensen TS. Ankle arthroplasty for rheumatoid arthritis and osteoarthritis: prospective long-term study of cemented replacements. J Bone Joint Surg Br 1998;80(2):328–32.

[26] Spirt AA, Assal M, Hansen ST Jr. Complications and failure after total ankle arthroplasty. J Bone Joint Surg Am 2004;86(6):1172–8.

[27] Kofoed H, Lundberg-Jensen A. Ankle arthroplasty in patients younger and older than 50 years: a prospective series with long-term follow-up. Foot Ankle Int 1999;20(8):501–6.

[28] Bjornadal L, Baecklund E, Yin L, et al. Decreasing mortality in patients with rheumatoid arthritis: results from a large population based cohort in Sweden, 1964–95. J Rheumatol 2002;29(5):906–12.

[29] Carlsson A, Markusson P, Sundberg M. Radiostereometric analysis of the double-coated STAR total ankle prosthesis: a 3–5 year follow-up of 5 cases with rheumatoid arthritis and 5 cases with osteoarthrosis. Acta Orthop 2005;76(4):573–9.

[30] Nishikawa M, Tomita T, Fujii M, et al. Total ankle replacement in rheumatoid arthritis. Int Orthop 2004;28(2):123–6.

[31] Shi K, Hayashida K, Hashimoto J, et al. Hydroxyapatite augmentation for bone atrophy in total ankle replacement in rheumatoid arthritis. J Foot Ankle Surg 2006;45(5):316–21.

[32] McGarvey WC, Clanton TO, Lunz D. Malleolar fracture after total ankle arthroplasty. Clin Orth Relat Res 2004;424:104–10.

[33] Myerson MS, Mroczek K. Perioperative complications of total ankle arthroplasty. Foot Ankle Int 2003;24(1):17–21.

[34] Kumar A, Dhar S. Total ankle replacement: early results during the learning period. Foot Ankle Surgery 2007;13:19–23.

[35] Haskell A, Mann RA. Perioperative complication rate of total ankle replacement is reduced by surgeon experience. Foot Ankle Int 2004;25(5):283–9.

ELSEVIER
SAUNDERS

Foot Ankle Clin N Am
12 (2007) 509–524

FOOT AND
ANKLE CLINICS

Wound Healing Complications and Infection Following Surgery for Rheumatoid Arthritis

Christopher Bibbo, DO, DPM, FACS, FAAOS, FACFAS

Department of Orthopedics, Marshfield Clinic, 1000 North Oak Avenue, Marshfield, WI 54449, USA

The patient who has rheumatoid arthritis (RA) often presents to foot and ankle specialists for the management of various musculoskeletal pathologies, often with crippling deformities of the forefoot, hindfoot, and ankle. Advances in the medical management of RA have allowed many patients to achieve previously unattainable levels of activity into later decades of life. This consequence from the improved medical management of RA is that although joint pain is being controlled from an inflammatory standpoint, musculoskeletal mechanical dysfunction that has already been incurred from years of low-grade, controlled disease continues unchecked. A perfect example of this is in the forefoot, in which multiple intrinsic and extrinsic musculoskeletal units are required for precise mechanical balance of the forefoot; despite good pain control and radiographic improvements in maintenance of bone mineral density, once biomechanical imbalances occur it is difficult, often impossible, to regain without ablative arthroplasties. Fortunately these surgical techniques have been shown to stand the test of time and to provide a platform for patients to regain functional ambulation. The foot and ankle surgeon, however, may be consulted to manage patients who have significant anatomic and biomechanical deformities, often in elderly, frail patients who depend on a host of disease-modifying medications. Additionally, even today there are still many areas of the nation that are underrepresented by rheumatologists, or patients are unable to access rheumatology services. In all these instances, patients may develop

E-mail address: bibbo.christopher@marshfieldclinic.org

1083-7515/07/$ - see front matter © 2007 Elsevier Inc. All rights reserved.
doi:10.1016/j.fcl.2007.04.005

severe deformities that impose more risk than usual for perioperative complications. The goal of the foot and ankle surgeon is to achieve balanced correction of deformity while minimizing the risk for complications. To achieve these goals, a large number of procedures may be required at a single or in a staged operative setting. In this article the evaluation of the patient who has RA to assess operative risks and the management of perioperative complications in the RA foot and ankle patient are presented.

Biologic considerations

Wound healing is multifactorial

Effect of age and gender

The aging process has been demonstrated clinically and experimentally to impair the healing process, with advancing age and male hormone status having a greater negative influence. Men and postmenopausal women demonstrate impaired collagen deposition and wound healing after surgical incisions [1,2]. Age-related elevated levels of thrombospondin 2, an inhibitor of angiogenesis, have also been experimentally linked to delayed wound healing [3]. The negative effect of age on wound healing is also attributable in part to a decrease in stem cell reserve and function associated with the aging process [4].

The preoperative evaluation of the patient who has rheumatoid arthritis

Cervical spine evaluation

Preoperative medical clearance is a necessity for patients who have RA undergoing major reconstructive foot and ankle surgery or in any patient undergoing general anesthesia, regardless of the extent of the intended operation. As part of the preoperative health screening process, all patients who have RA undergoing general anesthesia should be evaluated for cervical spine disease. An upper extremity and neurologic examination and screening C-spine radiograph (lateral flexion–extension films) uncover clinically significant C-spine rheumatoid disease. Positive findings should prompt neurosurgical evaluation and appropriate C-spine MRI studies. By this process the author has had the fortunate occurrence of twice in the past 5 years uncovering silent but alarming mechanical instability of the atlantoaxial junction. In both cases, successful neurosurgical management was followed by elective foot and ankle surgery.

Preoperative vascular evaluation

To minimize wound and infectious complications, before surgery the preoperative assessment of all patients must include a thorough vascular evaluation, arguably the most important evaluation as it relates to postoperative surgical site complications [5].

Arterial evaluation

Special attention is given to evaluation of the patient's arterial inflow status. The physical examination should include documentation of dorsalis pedis and posterior tibial pulses, capillary filling, and signs of venous insufficiency. Nonpalpable pedal pulses are an indication for noninvasive arterial studies, namely ankle–brachial indices (ABI). The author generally also reviews segmental limb pressures, because this information can key the clinician in to the anatomic location of arterial disease. A rule of thumb is that from one contiguous arterial segment to the next, there should not be a drop-off of more than 15 to 20 mm Hg pressure. When pulses are readily palpable further vascular evaluations are generally not required. A notable exception to this general rule is when the patient is a smoker and long-standing digital deformities are present. In these instances, when forefoot procedures are planned, it must be realized that distal to the arcuate artery, the caliber of the terminal arterial branches taper rapidly. Deformed toes fixed in place may now also have digital vessels fixed in position. Intimal changes, tunica media calcifications, and low-flow states place these toes at considerable risk. Surgical correction of the toe and simple manipulation of the toe at surgery may stretch the vessels past their tolerance, resulting in vascular embarrassment of the digit. Patients must be counseled as to the potential for digital vascular embarrassment after correction of long-standing toe deformities, which may result in simple tip necrosis to a frankly gangrenous toe. Preoperative evaluation by way of toe pressures and digital waveforms (pulse volume recordings) are helpful in establishing a baseline knowledge of toe vascularity and the potential for vascular embarrassment or healing complications. Toe pressures should be greater than 40 mm Hg for adequate healing, with pulsatile waveforms. Transcutaneous oximetry ($TcPO_2$) (transcutaneous oxygen measurements [TCOMs]) may also provide valuable information as to surgical wound healing potential. The author uses $TcPO_2$ when noninvasive arterial studies have proven suboptimal inflow and vascular reconstruction is not feasible. $TcPO_2$ values should generally be at greater than an absolute value of 40 mm Hg or a regional perfusion index (RPI) of 0.6 to ensure a high probability of healing. $TcPO_2$ values of 20 to 40 mm Hg or an RPI of 0.4 to 0.6 indicate an intermediate probability of healing; $TcPO_2$ values less than 20 mm Hg or an RPI less than 0.4 indicate a low probability of healing. Smokers are advised to quit smoking. Patients who have vasospastic disease are instructed to avoid all caffeinated beverages and foods in the perioperative period. In at-risk individuals, including patients who have marginal noninvasive studies, vasospastic disease, a subcutaneously tunneled arterial bypass, recent in situ lower extremity bypass (8 weeks), recent prosthetic graft leg bypass (8 weeks), or heavy smokers, a tourniquet during surgery is best avoided.

Venous evaluation

The venous examination, although less sophisticated, is helpful in determining which patients may develop delayed wound healing and persistent postoperative foot edema. The author simply searches for dependant rubor and signs of chronic venous stasis (history of ulceration, chronic skin pigmentation, and brawny induration) and performs a standing venous filling examination. Preoperatively edema control is achieved with Unna boots, compression stockings, or custom sequential compression devices. General skin conditioning is commenced with gentle emollients; treatment of localized dermatoses is used starting 3 to 4 weeks before surgery, up to the day of surgery, and postoperatively as needed. Psoriasis patients may harbor higher numbers of flora or even resistant flora; for these patients the author initiates daily washing of the part with chlorhexidine solution for 1 week before surgery. Patients who have severe psoriatic lesions are referred to dermatology before surgery.

Perioperative rheumatoid medications and complications

Steroids, methotrexate, D-penicillamine, cyclophosphamide, azathioprine, cyclosporine, leflunomide, nonsteroidal anti-inflammatory agents, and in particular, tumor necrosis-alpha (TNF-α) antagonists have all been implicated as causal agents for perioperative wound healing and infectious complications [6–9]. Because of the ever increasing role of the TNF-α antagonist in the medical management of RA, the impact of these agents on perioperative complications is explored in detail.

Effect of TNF-α inhibitors: basic science

TNF-α inhibitors have become more commonplace for the treatment of recalcitrant disease and the early management of RA. TNF-α is a ubiquitous 56-kD protein cytokine produced by endothelial cells, macrophages, and T-cells that is encoded on chromosome 6. TNF-α is an important mediator in the normal inflammatory cascade and is believed to be required for normal tissue healing and immune surveillance [7,10,11]. Several cell signaling pathways are believed to be involved with the TNF-α pathway. Recently the neutrophil activation antigen CD-69 has been found to be expressed at baseline in patients who have RA but reduced after TNF-α inhibitor therapy [12]. TNF-α inhibitor therapy has also been demonstrated to result in apoptosis of macrophage/monocyte lineage cells, which has also been suggested as a potential mechanism for inhibition of inflamed joint synovium in patients who have RA [13]. TNF-α antagonists have also been demonstrated to down-regulate the OPG/RANKL system of already TNF-primed osteocytes and endothelial cells [14]. These findings and others point to a complex array of functions that involve TNF-α. and the immune system. There is, however, no compelling basic science data demonstrating a certain and critical suppression of immune system function as it relates to the suppression of vital function of the neutrophil/macrophage system that would lead to an immune system left incompetent to survey and combat bacterial infections.

Numerous basic science investigations have demonstrated that the direct application to healing tissue [15–17] and the systemic administration of TNF-α during wound healing [18] result in a decrease in collagen production and wound strength by way of down-regulation of collagen gene expression [19]. These counterintuitive results regarding the inhibitory effect of TNF-α on wound collagen production are explained by experimental data demonstrating that the inhibitory effect of TNF-α is attenuated by the presence of an intact IL-1 counter-regulatory system [20].

Additionally, experimental data have shown that the binding of excess TNF-α by specific antibodies ameliorates the negative influence of TNF-α on wound healing [18,21].

Clinical studies

Examples of TNF-α antagonist medications used to treat patients who have RA include etanercept (Enbrel) and infliximab (Remicade). Etanercept is a recombinant soluble human TNF receptor that is covalently linked to a human IgG Fc fragment (p75 sTNFR:Fc fusion protein), which is administered subcutaneously twice a week. Infliximab is a chimeric human/mouse anti-TNF monoclonal antibody administered intravenously every 4 to 8 weeks. Both agents exert their main action by blocking the binding of synovial TNF-α to immunocompetent target cells, preventing the release of inflammatory mediators.

Clinically several reports warn of an increase in serious infections in patients receiving TNF-α antagonists [22,23]. Most notably a recent large British national prospective observational study of more than 7000 patients receiving TNF-α antagonist were compared with control patients who had RA in relation to the development of serious infections, defined as infection requiring hospitalization, intravenous antibiotics, or death. The investigators found that patients who had RA receiving TNF-α antagonists had a higher rate of serious infection; however, the overwhelming leading type of infection was lower respiratory. Causal organisms were mostly *Mycobacterium* spp., *Legionella pneumophila*, *Listeria monocytogenes*, and *Salmonella*. Bone and soft-tissue infections were 67% less common than respiratory infections. Urinary tract infections assumed a similar role as bone and soft tissue. Additionally, data specifically addressing the orthopedic surgery status among study patients was not provided [24]. Although these data underscore the potential severe nature of infection and TNF-α inhibition treatment, the types of infections seem to be predominantly intracellular lung infections, those of which that are not typical of a postoperative orthopedic infection after clean elective surgery.

To date only a few studies have specifically addressed complications in patients who have RA and the relationship of RA medications to complication rates. In the general orthopedic arthroplasty literature it has been clearly shown that methotrexate does not need to be discontinued before elective orthopedic surgery; in fact some investigators have noted lower infection rates in patients who have maintained their methotrexate regimen in the perioperative period [25,26]. Other investigations have not been able to discern an independent risk for perioperative joint arthroplasty wound and infectious complications based on RA medications [27]. Reports examining the affect of leflunomide on perioperative elective orthopedic surgery seem to be equivocal [28,29].

The literature specific to complications of RA foot and ankle surgery is limited to only a few studies. In 2003 Bibbo and colleagues [30] reported on complications in 104 patients who had RA who underwent clean, elective foot and ankle surgery. The investigators' study population underwent 725 procedures with an overall 32% complication rate. Wound healing problems were the most common complication, followed by superficial infections and delayed/nonunions; all complications were minor. Logistic regression analysis failed to reveal any statistical association between RA medications, age greater than 55 years, gender, number of procedures per patient, or presence of rheumatoid nodules, and the occurrence of healing or infectious complications. In this study, NSAIDs, steroids, methotrexate, hydroxychloroquine, and gold were the primary RA medications analyzed. In a follow-up study that specifically examined the effect of TNF-α antagonists on wound healing and infectious complications after foot and ankle surgery, Bibbo and Goldberg [10] prospectively followed patients undergoing clean, elective foot and ankle surgery for the development of complications in the postoperative period. Although the patient group who continued their TNF-α antagonists in the perioperative period had more smokers than the non-TNF-α group, fewer complications were seen in the TNF-α group ($P = .033$). Additionally this study did not find an increased risk for complications in those patients taking leflunomide. Although the study number was small (N = 33), these findings are important to consider in patients whose RA symptoms are disabling when their TNF-α antagonist medications are withheld. As a continuation of that database, the author currently has more than tripled the original study number; preliminary analysis of the expanded database reveals nearly identical results.

Other RA foot and ankle surgery studies have provided data on general complication rates (not specifically examining the influence of medications). Reize and colleagues [31] reported a 14% infection rate (equally distributed among superficial and deep) after metatarsal head resections. Anderson and colleagues [32] report a 4% nonunion and a 12% deep infection rate in patients who have RA undergoing tibiotalocalcaneal fusion with retrograde IM nailing. The same investigators reported only a 26% primary union rate for ankle fusions performed with compression screws [33]. These data are in stark contrast to those of Nagashima and colleagues [34], who reported a 100% union rate, a 0% infection rate, and a 24% wound complication rate for patients who had RA who underwent ankle fusion with a modified IM nail technique.

An important consideration in any surgical candidate is bacterial skin colonization. One unique study examined the bacterial carriage rate of patients who had RA receiving TNF-α antagonist therapy compared with control patients. The investigators demonstrated that the carriage rate of *Staphylococcus aureus* in patients who had RA on TNF-α inhibitors was not increased over control subjects [35]. This finding is of particular interest in light of the fact that the most common organism causing infection in patients who have RA undergoing orthpedic surgery is *S. aureus* [36].

Based on available data, the author's opinion at this time is thus that although there exists theoretic risks for perioperative complications associated with specific RA medications, the major risk for developing a postoperative wound or infectious complication seems to be more related to the inherent risk of the procedure, host fragility (inherent to RA?), and the genomic make-up of the host for healing, rather than the influence of a specific medication on a specific host's healing capability. When dealing with the issue of the perioperative management of RA medication in patients undergoing clean, elective foot and ankle surgery, the author uses a simple algorithm for the management of perioperative medications that is based on the available basic science of wound healing, the orthopedic literature, and the author's own current database on complications in RA foot and ankle patients.

For those patients undergoing clean, elective RA foot and ankle surgery (especially for those whose disease symptoms are overwhelming without their RA medications), the author does not require discontinuation of RA medications in the perioperative period. Notable exceptions include:

1. Patients who have a documented history of poor wound healing (in particular, methotrexate is held); these patients should have their medications held based on each individual drug half-life.
2. Patients who develop a postoperative infection or a wound-healing complication (in particular, methotrexate, steroids, TNF-α inhibitors, and IL-1 inhibitors are held); medications may be resumed after wounds are healed or infections cleared.
3. When operating on patients referred for infection, these medications are withheld immediately and resumed as outlined (Table 1).

A special mention should be made as to those patients who have RA who pose a triple threat for complications: patients who have RA who smoke, drink, and have poorly controlled type I diabetes (as measured by HbA1c). This subset of patients who have RA is a challenge, and a conservative, individualized approach must be taken to their perioperative

Table 1
When to consider the perioperative discontinuation of RA medications

- Documented history of poor wound healing
- Documented history of same-site infection requiring long-term antibiotics
- Active same-site infection/remote infection
- Active same-site poor wound healing
- Patient is at risk for poor healing:
  Total protein less >3.5 g/dL
  Total lymphocyte count >1500/mL
  Abnormally low transferrin, prealbumin, retinol binding protein levels
  Elevated hemoglobin A-1c (patients who have diabetes)
  Abnormally low cholesterol levels (elderly patients)
- Difficult revision surgery:
  Anticipated prolonged tourniquet time (>2 h)
  Dissection through difficult scars and devitalized planes
  Extensive soft-tissue stripping
- Multiple RA medications + smoking + alcohol abuse + elevated HbA1c

medication plan. Additionally, more frequent postoperative follow-up than usual is recommended (every 1–2 weeks until healed).

Acute deformity correction and impact on complications

Patients presenting with long-standing deformities present the risk for complications stemming from lack of tissue pliability from being in a chronically deformed state. This is particularly important when considering surgical correction of toe deformities. Over time, hammer and claw toes become ever more rigid; metatarsophalangeal joint subluxation proceeds to dorsal dislocation. With this process, the digital vessels match the deformity and assume a shortened position. Acute toe correction with straightening temporarily either stretches or buckles the vessel, narrowing the lumen and potentially injuring the intima. Intimal injury may lead to vessel thrombosis, placing the toes at risk for relative irreversible critical ischemia or venous impairment. Power saw vibrations may also set the stage for acute vessel spasm and vascular embarrassment. Surgeons who perform a large volume of RA cases in their career have almost uniformly experienced digital ischemia or venous engorgement after RA toe surgery. To prevent permanent ischemic changes, it is incumbent on the surgeon to quickly implement measures to reverse the problem (Figs. 1 and 2).

Another major consequence of acutely correcting a chronic deformity in the patient who has RA includes difficulties in wound closure and healing. This becomes important when straight incisions are placed over concave surfaces (contracted skin) or when angular corrections (lengthening) are performed acutely within a chronically shortened segment. This may lead to an inability to close incisions, excessive skin tension and subsequent necrosis of

Intra-Operative Management of Blue Toe (Venous Insult)

Warm saline sponge to toe (do not let toe get cold)
↓
Infiltrate 1% lidocaine plain to operative site
↓
Continue warm saline sponge covering toe
↓
Ensure no local tourniquet effect
↓
Remove pin & reposition to lesser degree of correction
↓
Permanently remove pin, allow toe to assume position of pre-op deformity
↓
Start low dose heparin drip (500-800 units/hour) & continue postoperatively
↓
Loosen post-op dressings
↓
Elevate to level of bed only; no ice; caffeine-free diet
↓
Baby ASA PO QD; no smoking; no nicotine patches
↓
Physical Therapy: no dependency longer than 10-15 minutes
↓
D/C on Lovenox 40mg SC QD or baby ASA & above dietary/social restrictions
↓
Follow progress weekly; most resolve over 3-4 weeks

Fig. 1. Intraoperative management of blue toe (venous insult).

incisions, and de novo skin breakdown on areas in which incisions have not been placed. In these instances, careful planning of incision placement (eg, plantar approach to metatarsal heads) and the availability of back-up plans for wound closure (eg, VAC, local tissue rotations) are paramount. In instances in which acute correction places the skin at risk, it is often best to provide relief of length (ie, shorten instead of lengthening) to maintain the integrity of the soft-tissue envelop.

Intraoperative measures to prevent complications

Routine preoperative prophylactic antibiotics are used, typically a first-generation cephalosporin such as cefazolin (modified from [5]). When patients are penicillin/cephalosporin allergic, clindamycin (900 mg) or levofloxacin (500 mg) are used in the perioperative period. Vancomycin is used for patients who have a history of MRSA colonization (and a documented lack of eradication of such colonization). Patients who have RA and who

Intra-Operative Management of Pale Toe (Arterial Insult)

Immediately remove pin & reposition to lesser degree of correction

↓

Immediately infiltrate 1% lidocaine plain to operative site

↓

Warm saline sponge to toe (do not let toe get cold)

↓

Continue warm saline sponge covering toe

↓

Have anesthesia elevate patient blood pressure to normotensive level

↓

Ensure no local tourniquet effect

↓

If toe "pinks-up", resume case
Re-consider the use of power saw, & use smaller diameter pins, or no pins

Toe remains pale?

↓

Check digital Doppler signals intra-op

↓

Repeat above maneuvers: if no Doppler signals, or no bleeding from tissues,
finish case as quickly as possible

↓

Repeat digital arterial exam in recovery (CFT, Doppler, pulse oximetry)

↓

Vascular consult to rule-out embolic phenomenon from proximal vessel disease?

↓

Keep foot warm; check post-op pulse oximetry

↓

Start low dose heparin drip (500-800 units/hour); continue post-op until d/c

↓

Baby ASA PO QD; no smoking; no nicotine patches

↓

Elevate to level of bed only; no ice; caffeine-free diet

Recalcitrant Arterial Insult ?

↓

Intra-arterial streptokinase (?)

↓

Microvascular repair (????)

Fig. 2. Intraoperative management of pale toe (arterial insult).

are on steroids often possess thin, fragile skin, with only a thin layer of subcutaneous tissue. Delicate, atraumatic operative techniques must be used. Tourniquet use should be limited in these at-risk patients, but when a tourniquet must be used, the total tourniquet time should never exceed

120 minutes. The lowest pressure setting to provide visualization is used; a pressure of 125 points above the systolic provides adequate hemostasis for visualization of the operative field. Often in thin-skinned patients and elderly patients a tourniquet should not be used. When moving to a second operative site during surgery (eg, harvesting iliac crest bone graft), the limb tourniquet should be released and the foot/ankle wounds packed and wrapped with gentle compression (sterile Coban or an Esmarch works well). When returning to the main operative field, the surgeon often finds that bleeding is well controlled and tourniquet reinflation is not required.

In those patients on anticoagulants and antiplatelet agents, steps should be taken to minimize hematoma formation. The author does not require that patients discontinue Coumadin or Plavix (clopidogrel) before elective surgery; often the risks of discontinuing therapeutic anticoagulation outweigh the risks of the effect on hemostasis. The tourniquet should be released before subcutaneous closure and bleeding assessed. When general anesthesia is used, relative hypotension is common. The reduced limb perfusion pressure may give the false impression of controlled hemostasis. A systolic pressure of approximately 95 mm Hg is required for a femoral pulse, with incrementally higher inflow pressures required to adequately fill more distal arterial segments. In these instances the anesthesia staff should be instructed to bring the blood pressure to greater than 100 to 110 mm Hg systolic, which can be done by lightening-up the patients (vasopressors are not needed) and hemostasis reassessed. Packing the wound with Gelfoam and applying a pressure wrap for 5 to 10 minutes controls most bleeding. When surgical bleeding from a broad surface does not respond to cautery/suture or pressure, a slurry of Gelfoam and thrombin (1 g powdered Gelfoam + thrombin 1000 U in 10 ml sterile saline for injection) applied into the operative field with an overlying pressure bandage is helpful to control bleeding. Persistent brisk bleeding beyond this may require checking the aPTT/PT-INR and infusion of fresh frozen plasma.

This same approach can be helpful in instances in which digital perfusion is questionable after placement of retrograde pins. When digital inflow is in question, the first step is to monitor the response to an elevation in blood pressure. Warming the digits with warm saline-soaked gauze on the toes and at the ankle may assist in breaking an episode of vasospasm. Creating a relative shortening of the digit by sliding the toe up the pin can take off any excess stretch of digital vessels. The local application of nitroglycerin ointment or intra-arterial lidocaine is rarely needed. Ultimately the author has found that an unresponsive toe requires pin removal. Once a toe pin is removed for this reason it should not be replaced, because the original problem most often recurs. Local application of lidocaine to the operative field may be helpful if vasospasm or venous engorgement persists. Postoperative venous engorgement of a toe is treated best with elevation and observation. If cyanosis persists, the pin is removed. Postoperatively the limb is rested at heart level and ice is avoided. Smoking, nicotine patches, and caffeine are restricted. In most instances, careful observation results in a good outcome (Table 1). Simple digital tip necrosis usually results in an acceptable cosmetic and functional result. The surgeons must counsel the patients before surgery of these potential complications.

Immediate postoperative course

Antibiotics are used for 24 to 36 hours postoperatively. Drains are generally removed in 24 hours (modified from [5]). Edema control is balanced with positioning of the foot for optimal perfusion. Elevation is generally acceptable at two-pillow height. It may be best to avoid the application of ice after digital cases, especially when concern exists for the vascular status of the part. Caffeine and all nicotine products are restricted. Supplemental oxygen therapy is considered in at-risk toes, when flaps are created, and when susceptible incisions are created, such as incisions used for the approach for total ankle arthroplasty. Nasal cannula oxygen may be uncomfortable for the patients, thus humidified oxygen may provide better patient compliance (eg, 50%–100% humidified face mask O_2 for 24 h). Ambulation with assistance/physical therapy is begun as soon as possible. Postoperative nausea may be a significant hindrance to patient recuperation after general anesthesia, especially in elderly patients and those who have gastrointestinal dysmotility. Antiemetics are effective, especially when coupled with promotility agents.

Pain control

Pain control is paramount for patient comfort and to promote progression in physical therapy (modified from [5]). Regional anesthesia provides excellent postoperative pain relief during the immediate postoperative period and may be continued after discharge through the use of outpatient indwelling regional nerve sheath catheters. In addition to regional anesthesia modalities, patient-controlled analgesia (narcotics) should be implemented for postoperative pain control after large reconstructions. NSAIDs (eg, parenteral Toradol) are administered as a scheduled supplement for the first 24 to 36 hours. The author's observation has been that the short-term use of NSAIDs does not adversely affect soft-tissue or bony healing. Long-acting oral opioids with rescue dosing (eg, OxyContin, 10–20 mg orally every 12 h plus OxyIR, 5 mg orally every 4–6 h as needed for break-though pain) may be started on postoperative day number 1. The author continues this regimen for up to 2 weeks and then transitions to shorter duration agents (eg, Vicodin) thereafter. In most instances, with early aggressive pain control, narcotic use may be discontinued after 3 weeks. Intramuscular medications should be avoided in patients being actively anticoagulated.

Deep vein thrombosis prophylaxis

Although RA does not impart a higher risk than the general population for the development of a deep venous thrombosis (DVT), these patients may quickly become sedentary after lower extremity orthopedic surgery and thus may be considered at-risk for DVT from a functional standpoint (modified from [5]). Rheumatic diseases may coexist in patients, and other rheumatic disorders, such as systemic lupus, carry a higher risk for DVT. All patients have compression stockings on the unaffected limb, preferably commencing in the operating room. It is the author's practice to place all patients who have RA who will be non-weightbearing on unfractionated heparin (eg, Lovenox, 30 mg SQ every 12 h or 40 mg SQ daily) within 24 hours postoperatively while in the hospital. Patients continue daily dosing (eg, Lovenox, 40 mg SQ daily) for 2 to 3 weeks on discharge from the hospital. Outpatients are generally undergoing procedures that allow full or partial weightbearing, and for patients who have no prior history of a DVT a daily baby ASA for 2 to 3 weeks has proven adequate in this setting. Any patient who is actively anticoagulated or is undergoing antiplatelet therapy (ASA, clopidogrel) has their medication resumed immediately postoperatively. Patients on warfarin with therapeutic target INRs of ≥ 3 are started on unfractionated heparin, which is resumed immediately postoperatively to a therapeutic aPTT while their warfarin is resumed until their target INR is reached.

Any patient who presents in the postoperative period with clinical signs and symptoms of a DVT should undergo lower extremity duplex scanning. Scans positive for a DVT in the deep femoral–popliteal system are begun on immediate anticoagulation with either full-dose fractionated heparin or unfractionated heparin with transition to warfarin. Heparin therapy for at least 36 hours has been believed to assist in decreasing vessel wall inflammation. Oral anticoagulation should be continued for 3 to 6 months. Acute thrombosis in the calf veins that are within 2 cm of the popliteal system or in the saphenous system within 2 cm of the fossa ovalis should be considered for therapeutic anticoagulation. The author has observed that these thromboses tend to propagate more readily into the deep venous system. Otherwise calf vein involvement may be reasonably treated with ASA with repeat scanning at 2-week intervals to assess for clot propagation. Propagation of calf thrombi should be managed as a deep thrombosis, especially in prothrombotic populations. Symptomatic treatment of minor thrombosis includes elevation, warm moist heat, and oral NSAIDs.

Subacute postoperative considerations

Suture removal

Postoperative edema on an extremity with multiple skin incisions paints a clear picture that illustrates a need for ample time for wound healing, especially in postmenopausal women and in men [1,2] (modified from [5]). The author therefore does not rush to remove sutures; sutures or staples may need to be left in place for up to 4 to 6 weeks or more until edema and wounds are adequately healed. To minimize the risk for pin-track infections, however, percutaneous pins should be removed as soon as possible, usually at 4 to 6 weeks. Pins that have backed out should never be reinserted. Patients should be instructed to tape in place in the extruded position any pin that has backed out and immediately notify the surgeon, especially if pain, erythema, and swelling occur.

Edema and hematoma management

During the postoperative course, edema is universal. TCOMs on edematous feet show decreases in oxygen tensions (modified from [5]). Excess interstitial fluid finds portals for exit and tends to perpetuate a situation of chronic seepage of fluid through pin tracts and incisions, a set-up for bacterial colonization and infection. Edema control enhances wound healing and relieves discomfort from excess interstitial fluid. In certain patients effective edema control may be difficult. Strict elevation, and when wounds have epithelialized, edema wraps (Unna boot, elastic wraps), however, are usually effective in controlling most localized edema. If edema fluid is found to be leaking through unhealed incisions and pin tracts, antibiotics may be added for a short course. Elderly patients who demonstrate new bilateral edema postoperatively should be suspect for fluid retention of renal/cardiac origin and referred to their primary care provider. In these instances, appropriate diuresis may assist in edema control. When surgical corrections are stable, compression garments used for 1 to 2 months postoperatively are of great benefit. Compression garments should impart 20 to 30 mm Hg of pressure for typical postoperative edema.

Patients who are anticoagulated may develop postoperative subcutaneous hematomas. If large, these may be aspirated early if incisions or the overlying skin is in jeopardy, or these may be aspirated late (during liquefaction before resorption). Patients who have RA are prone to infectious complications, whether on steroids or not, with increased mortality from infection. The author therefore does not hesitate to administer a short course (7–10 days) of prophylactic antibiotics (eg, Keflex, 500 mg orally once daily) in patients who have a hematoma or continued serous drainage, especially if a low-grade fever, pain, or erythema is present. Frankly cellulitic areas overlying a suspected hematoma warrant consideration for urgent irrigation, debridement, cultures, and sensitivities. At this stage debridement may be minimal, with preservation of soft tissues. Left ignored, a simple complication may result in a large abscess area capable of compressing and rapidly thrombosing small vessels and producing widespread deep necrosis. In patients on active anticoagulation presenting with an unusually large hematoma, surgical evacuation of the hematoma and evaluation of the patient's coagulation profiles (aPTT/PTT-INR) should ensue.

References

[1] Engeland CG, Bosch JA, Cacioppo JT, et al. Mucosal wound healing: the roles of age and sex. Arch Surg 2006;141(12):1193–7.

[2] Lenhardt R, Hopf HW, Marker E, et al. Perioperative collagen deposition in elderly and young men and women. Arch Surg 2000;135(1):71–4.

[3] Agah A, Kyriakides TR, Letrondo N, et al. Thrombospondin 2 levels are increased in aged mice: consequences for cutaneous wound healing and angiogenesis. Matrix Biol 2004;22(7): 539–47.

[4] Roh C, Lyle S. Cutaneous stem cells and wound healing. Pediatr Res 2006;59(4 Pt 2): 100R–3R.

[5] Bibbo C. The assessment and perioperative management of patients with rheumatoid arthritis. Techniques in Foot & Ankle Surgery 2004;3:126–35.

[6] Gorman JD, Sack KE, Davis JC Jr. Treatment of ankylosing spondylitis by inhibition of tumor necrosis factor alpha. N Engl J Med 2002;346:1349–56.

[7] Moreland LW, Bucy RP, Weinblatt ME, et al. Immune function in patients with rheumatoid arthritis treated with etanercept. Clin Immunol 2002;103:13–21.

[8] Weinblatt ME, Kremer JM, Bankhurst AD, et al. A trial of etanercept, a recombinant tumor necrosis factor receptor:Fc fusion protein, in patients with rheumatoid arthritis receiving methotrexate. N Engl J Med 1999;340:253–9.

[9] Yazici Y, Erkan D, Lockshin MD. A preliminary study of etanercept in the treatment of severe resistant psoriatic arthritis. Clin Exp Rheumatol 2000;18:732–4.

[10] Bibbo C, Goldberg JW. Infectious and healing complications after elective orthopaedic foot and ankle surgery during tumor necrosis factor-alpha inhibition therapy. Foot Ankle Int 2004;25(5):331–5.

[11] Alldred A. Etanercept in rheumatoid arthritis. Expert Opin Pharmacother 2001;7:1137–48.

[12] Capsoni F, Sarzi-Puttini P, Atzeni F, et al. Effect of adalimumab on neutrophil function in patients with rheumatoid arthritis. Arthritis Res Ther 2005;7:R250–5.

[13] Catrina AI, Trollmo C, af Klint E, et al. Evidence that anti-tumor necrosis factor therapy with both etanercept and infliximab induces apoptosis in macrophages, but not lymphocytes, in rheumatoid arthritis joints: extended report. Arthritis Rheum 2005;52(1):61–72.

[14] Catrina AI, af Klint E, Ernestam S, et al. Anti-tumor necrosis factor therapy increases synovial osteoprotegerin expression in rheumatoid arthritis. Arthritis Rheum 2006;54(1):76–81.

[15] Rapala K. The effect of tumor necrosis factor-alpha on wound healing. An experimental study. Ann Chir Gynaecol Suppl 1996;211:1–53.

[16] Rapala K, Laato M, Niinikoski J, et al. Tumor necrosis factor alpha inhibits wound healing in the rat. Eur Surg Res 1991;23(5–6):261–8.

[17] Rapala KT, Vaha-Kreula MO, Heino JJ, et al. Tumor necrosis factor-alpha inhibits collagen synthesis in human and rat granulation tissue fibroblasts. Experientia 1996;52(1):70–4.

[18] Lee RH, Efron DT, Tantry U, et al. Inhibition of tumor necrosis factor-alpha attenuates wound breaking strength in rats. Wound Repair Regen 2000;8(6):547–53.

[19] Rapala K, Peltonen J, Heino J, et al. Tumour necrosis factor-alpha selectively modulates expression of collagen genes in rat granulation tissue. Eur J Surg 1997;163(3):207–14.

[20] Maish GO 3rd, Shumate ML, Ehrlich HP, et al. Interleukin-1 receptor antagonist attenuates tumor necrosis factor-induced alterations in wound breaking strength. J Trauma 1999;47(3): 533–7.

[21] Regan MC, Kirk SJ, Hurson M, et al. Tumor necrosis factor-alpha inhibits in vivo collagen synthesis. Surgery 1993;113(2):173–7.

[22] Bongartz T, Sutton AJ, Sweeting MJ, et al. Anti-TNF antibody therapy in rheumatoid arthritis and the risk of serious infections and malignancies: systematic review and meta-analysis of rare harmful effects in randomized controlled trials. JAMA 2006;295(19):2275–85.

[23] Listing J, Strangfeld A, Kary S, et al. Infections in patients with rheumatoid arthritis treated with biologic agents. Arthritis Rheum 2005;52(11):3403–12.

[24] Dixon WG, Watson K, Lunt M, et al. British Society for Rheumatology Biologics Register. Rates of serious infection, including site-specific and bacterial intracellular infection, in rheumatoid arthritis patients receiving anti-tumor necrosis factor therapy: results from the British Society for Rheumatology Biologics Register. Arthritis Rheum 2006;54(8):2368–76.

[25] Grennan DM, Gray J, Loudon J, et al. Methotrexate and early postoperative complications in patients with rheumatoid arthritis undergoing elective orthopaedic surgery. Ann Rheum Dis 2001;60(3):214–7.

[26] Perhala RS, Wilke WS, Clough JD, et al. Local infectious complications following large joint replacement in rheumatoid arthritis patients treated with methotrexate versus those not treated with methotrexate. Arthritis Rheum 1991;34:146–52.

[27] Escalante A, Beardmore TD. Risk factors for early wound complications after orthopedic surgery for rheumatoid arthritis. J Rheumatol 1995;22:1844–51.

[28] Tanaka N, Sakahashi H, Sato E, et al. Examination of the risk of continuous leflunomide treatment on the incidence of infectious complications after joint arthroplasty in patients with rheumatoid arthritis. J Clin Rheumatol 2003;9:115–8.

[29] Fuerst M, Mohl H, Baumgartel K, et al. Leflunomide increases the risk of early healing complications in patients with rheumatoid arthritis undergoing elective orthopedic surgery. Rheumatol Int 2006;26:1138–42.

[30] Bibbo C, Anderson RB, Davis WH, et al. The influence of rheumatoid chemotherapy, age, and presence of rheumatoid nodules on postoperative complications in rheumatoid foot and ankle surgery: analysis of 725 procedures in 104 patients. Foot Ankle Int 2003;24(1):40–4.

[31] Reize P, Ina Leichtle C, Leichtle UG, et al. Long-term results after metatarsal head resection in the treatment of rheumatoid arthritis. Foot Ankle Int 2006;27:586–90.

[32] Anderson T, Linder L, Rydholm U, et al. Tibio-talocalcaneal arthrodesis as a primary procedure using a retrograde intramedullary nail: a retrospective study of 26 patients with rheumatoid arthritis. Acta Orthop 2005;76:580–7.

[33] Anderson T, Maxander P, Rydholm U, et al. Ankle arthrodesis by compression screws in rheumatoid arthritis: primary union in 9/35 patients. Acta Orthop 2005;76:884–90.

[34] Nagashima M, Tachihara A, Matsuzaki T, et al. Follow-up of ankle arthrodesis in severe hind foot deformity in patients with rheumatoid arthritis using an intramedullary nail with fins. Mod Rheumatol 2005;15:269–74.

[35] Bassettei S, Wasmer S, Hasler P, et al. *Staphylococcus aureus* in patients with rheumatoid arthritis under conventional and anti-tumor necrosis factor-alpha treatment. J Rheumatol 2005;32:2125–9.

[36] Barbari EF, Osmon DR, Duffy MC, et al. Outcome of prosthetic joint infection in patients with rheumatoid arthritis: the impact of medical and surgical therapy in 200 patients. Clin Infect Dis 2006;42:216–23.

ELSEVIER
SAUNDERS

Foot Ankle Clin N Am
12 (2007) 525–537

FOOT AND
ANKLE CLINICS

Rheumatoid Arthritis

Marlyn Lorenzo, MD, FACR

Mercy Medical Center, 301 St. Paul Place, Suite 411, Baltimore, MD 21202

Rheumatoid arthritis (RA) is a chronic systemic autoimmune connective tissue disorder that primarily targets the joints, specifically the synovial membranes, causing inflammatory arthritis. The disease affects all ethnic groups and has a prevalence of approximately 1%. It affects predominantly women, with a women-to-men ratio of 2:1 and a peak incidence between the ages of 40 and 60 years. Individuals affected by the disease are genetically predisposed, and it is believed that there is an environmental exposure or exogenous event that precipitates the disease. The pathology of the disease as it targets the joints is initiated by infiltration of the synovial membrane by inflammatory cells, predominantly T-cells and macrophages. Synovial hyperplasia and angiogenesis result from this injury to the synovial membrane. This inflammatory process that occurs in the synovial membrane is expanded and extends into the adjacent cartilage and bone, leading to the destruction of these, characterized by loss of articular cartilage and eventually periarticular bone erosions [1].

Approximately 85% of patients who have the disease are rheumatoid factor positive. Rheumatoid factor is an antibody directed against the Fc portion of immunoglobulin G (IgG). Even though it is not present in all patients who have RA, it is believed that when it is, it has a role in the disease process. Immune complexes with rheumatoid factor have been shown in patients who have RA, and one theory is that it is possible that these activate the complement cascade contributing to the inflammatory process in RA, although there is no definite proof for this. There is also an antibody directed against cyclic citrullinated peptide (anti-CCP antibody) that has recent use as part of the diagnostic process in RA and that has been shown to be more specific for RA than the rheumatoid factor [1–5]. Also of note, approximately 30% of patients who have RA can have a positive antinuclear antibody (ANA).

1083-7515/07/$ - see front matter © 2007 Elsevier Inc. All rights reserved.
doi:10.1016/j.fcl.2007.04.004

Diagnosis

There is no specific test available that can determine whether someone has RA. The diagnosis is made by a combination of findings that are obtained through history, physical examination, and laboratory and radiographic data. A set of criteria therefore was developed and revised by The American Rheumatism Association in 1987 [6]. These criteria include morning stiffness lasting at least 1 hour, soft-tissue swelling or fluid in at least three joint areas simultaneously observed by a physician, at least one area swollen in a wrist, metacarpophalangeal (MCP), or proximal interphalangeal (PIP) joint, symmetric arthritis (without absolute symmetry is acceptable), rheumatoid nodules, abnormal amounts of serum rheumatoid factor, and erosions or bony decalcification on radiographs of the hand and wrist. A diagnosis is considered when four of these criteria are present; if only the first three are present, they should be present for at least 6 weeks.

There are multiple differential diagnoses to consider when considering a diagnosis of RA. Some of these include other connective tissue disorders like lupus or Sjögren' syndrome; infectious etiologies, including viral arthritides and less likely bacterial; crystal-induced arthritis, including gout and pseudogout; seronegative arthropathies, including psoriatic and reactive arthritis; paraneoplastic syndromes, sarcoidosis, osteoarthritis, hypothyroidism, and fibromyalgia.

Patients who have RA can have variable presentations of the disease. For example, a patient can present with a sudden onset of a symmetric polyarthritis, in which case other causes of acute polyarthritis, particularly infectious etiologies, should be excluded first. A more common presentation is a more gradual onset of symptoms that can begin with arthralgias, generalized malaise, fevers, decreased appetite, and then the arthritis. Less often it could have a monoarticular onset, and here also, other etiologies must be excluded first. The latter might be a cause for delay in diagnosis, because it does not follow the classic presentation and therefore it is difficult to establish the diagnosis early on, but rather when the disease has progressed to a more classic presentation. If left untreated, RA usually progresses and leads to structural damage and joint deformity, and it has the potential to ultimately cause severe disability in many cases.

Parameters to assess disease severity

Multiple therapies are currently available for the treatment of RA. In recent years a significant number of US Food and Drug Administration (FDA) approvals have emerged as new treatment alternatives for RA. Some of these, for example rituximab, are medications that have been on the market for many years but have not been looked into with more detail as therapeutic targets for RA until recently, based on new insights into the disease pathogenesis. When choosing the right medication to use in patients who have RA, one has to consider each patient and assess them individually, taking into account different aspects of the disease, including disease severity or activity and comorbidities. The more aggressive the disease, the more aggressive one has to be with the management. There are different parameters available to measure disease activity that could be used in clinical practice to help clinicians have an objective way of measuring disease severity and guide therapy. These include the Disease Activity Score (DAS), the DAS28 score, which is a modification of the DAS, and the Simplified Disease Activity Index (SDAI). The assessment of physical function can be measured separately using the Health Assessment Questionnaire.

In general practice, one often looks at these parameters separately before deciding which therapy is best in a particular case. Some of these include whether the patient has seropositive or seronegative disease, presence of synovitis or soft-tissue swelling, pain assessed by the visual analog scale (VAS), rheumatoid nodules, erosive changes or definite periarticular osteopenia on radiographs, elevated markers of inflammation, including sedimentation rate and C-reactive protein, and even anemia of inflammation if this is secondary to the arthritis. Other parameters include number of joints involved and duration of morning stiffness. Besides these parameters that look predominantly at joint disease, in determining the severity of the disease one needs to consider whether there are extra-articular manifestations of the disease. Some of the extra-articular manifestations in RA include interstitial lung disease, pericarditis, ophthalmologic disease (most commonly scleritis), and vasculitis. Patients who have seropositive disease are more likely to develop extra-articular manifestations than patients who have seronegative disease. The presence of extra-articular manifestations is by itself a marker of disease severity and therefore an indication that aggressive therapy should be considered.

Algorithm for selection of drug therapy in rheumatoid arthritis

Available therapies include nonsteroidal anti-inflammatories, corticosteroids, and disease-modifying antirheumatic drugs (DMARDs). The disease-modifying drugs currently used most commonly include sulfasalazine (SSA), antimalarials (particularly hydroxychloroquine), methotrexate (MTX), and tumor necrosis factor (TNF)-inhibitors. TNF inhibitors, abatacept and rituximab are colloquially known as biologic DMARDs or simply as biologics. More recently approved therapies for RA include abatacept and rituximab. There are other therapies available used less frequently, and those include leflunomide (Arava), gold, anakinra (IL-1 inhibitor), minocycline, D-penicillamine, azathioprine, and cyclosporine. Cyclophosphamide has been used mainly for extra-articular manifestations of the disease, particularly vasculitis. Anti-inflammatories are used mainly for pain control but are not considered adequate as solo therapy for RA, because there is no evidence that these prevent disease progression. This is usually an alternative initial therapy if a patient presents with symptoms suggestive of RA but has not yet undergone a complete evaluation; oral corticosteroids are also used in this setting if there is significant synovitis or if anti-inflammatories have already been used with an inadequate response. Once the diagnosis of RA is made, however, other treatment alternatives should be considered. It is common practice among rheumatologists to use corticosteroids at the beginning of therapy. These are usually used in a low dose, which is effective in most cases and can provide significant clinical improvement in a short period of time, giving time for the disease-modifying agents to begin working. The goal is usually to discontinue the corticosteroids once the disease is controlled by the chosen disease-modifying drug. Next comes the big question: Which disease-modifying therapy should one choose from all of the available alternatives? After taking into consideration the aforementioned aspects of the disease in each individual patient, even though there is no specific rule, in general a possible approach would be the following. For mild seronegative RA with no evidence of erosive disease, hydroxychloroquine or SSA would be an adequate starting treatment alternative. Hydroxychloroquine is the drug with the safest side-effect profile. There is a risk for retinopathy that could lead to visual loss and that can occur within several months to several years after initiation of daily therapy. For this reason, every patient who is to begin therapy with hydroxychloroquine should have a baseline ophthalmologic examination and repeat examinations at least every 6 months to 1 year thereafter, even though the manufacturer's recommendation is to have an ophthalmologic examination every 3 months. For SSA, because of the risks for bone marrow suppression and elevation of liver enzymes, these patients require regular monitoring of these and occasionally of their renal function also [7]. If the patient does not improve on these drugs or if there is more aggressive disease manifested by seropositive disease, significantly elevated markers of inflammation, and more extensive clinical disease, MTX would then be a good choice. If it is used in a patient who had a partial response to hydroxychloroquine or SSA, then MTX could be added to the regimen; otherwise it should be used as monotherapy. The usual starting dose of MTX is 7.5 mg per week, which can be titrated up to 20 mg weekly if oral or 25 mg weekly if administered parenterally. As with SSA, MTX therapy requires regular blood tests to assess for side effects [8,9]. In a randomized study published in *Arthritis and Rheumatism* in 2002, the efficacy of combination therapy with these three medications was compared [10]. Patients were randomized to receive a combination of MTX with hydroxychloroquine, MTX with SSA, or a combination of MTX, SSA, and hydroxychloroquine. Results of this study showed a better efficacy using triple combination therapy, with a statistically significant difference in patients achieving American College of Rheumatology (ACR) 20%, 50%, and 70% responses, respectively. Patients enrolled in this study all had evidence of active disease. The parameters to measure active disease in this study included erythrocyte sedimentation rate (ESR), the presence of morning stiffness, and tender and swollen joint count. Based on this study, triple combination therapy is therefore an effective and well-tolerated combination that could be used in patients who have active RA. A similar study published in 1996 in the *New England Journal of Medicine* compared this combination of triple therapy to MTX alone and to a combination of SSA and hydroxychloroquine [11]. This study also showed that triple therapy was superior to either MTX alone or a combination of SSA and hydroxychloroquine.

Mechanism of action of antirheumatic drugs

In terms of mechanism of action (MOA) of antirheumatic drugs, the basic underlying common denominator is that they affect the inflammatory cascade involved in the pathogenesis of RA, each at different levels (even though the levels are not well established for all of them). For example, MTX is a folic acid analog, also called a folate antimetabolite, that inhibits the enzyme dihydrofolate reductase, blocking the production of its active metabolite, folinic acid. This causes a blockage of the folinic acid-dependent pathways, including purine and pyrimidine metabolism, which leads to the synthesis of purines [9]. Similarly, leflunomide (Arava) works as a pyrimidine synthesis inhibitor, and this is its proposed mechanism of action in RA. Despite these similarities, it is not clear if the main MOA of MTX is through this pathway or from a combination of actions. MTX increases the release of adenosine, and studies have shown that adenosine is an important mediator of inflammation. In an animal study using adenosine receptor-deficient mice, it was shown that mice that did not have these receptors did not have a reduction in inflammatory mediators, including leukocytes and TNF-α, while on MTX therapy [12,13].

Biologics

Another alternative in patients who have more active and aggressive disease are the TNF-inhibitors. These should be considered when there is no response or partial response to the DMARDs discussed earlier and can be used as monotherapy or in combination with other DMARDs. Studies have shown that TNF-inhibitors are more efficacious when used in combination with MTX therapy. There are three available TNF-inhibitors on the market. These include etanercept (Enbrel), adalimumab (Humira), and infliximab (Remicade) [14–33]. All of them block TNF-α activity. Etanercept was the first one approved in 1998 as therapy for RA. It is a fusion protein that works by binding soluble TNF-α and -β. In contrast, adalimumab and infliximab are monoclonal antibodies that bind soluble and cellbound TNF-α but not TNF-β. Even though adalimumab and infliximab are both monoclonal antibodies, adalimumab is a fully human monoclonal antibody, whereas Remicade is a chimeric mouse–human monoclonal antibody and has been associated with the development of antibodies called human anti-chimeric antibodies, or HACA. Etanercept has been associated with the development of non-neutralizing antibodies to the TNF-receptor portion or other protein components of the drug product. No apparent correlation of antibody development to clinical response or adverse events has been observed. Other important differences between these include their routes of administration and their half-lives. Etanercept and adalimumab are administered subcutaneously every week or every other week, respectively; Remicade is administered as an intravenous infusion every 8 weeks after induction therapy.

Abatacept (Orencia) became available on the market in February of 2006. It is a cytotoxic human T-lymphocyte–associated antigen 4 (CTLA-4) immunoglobulin (Ig), or CTLA4 Ig that binds to CD80 and CD86 (present on antigen-presenting cells), blocking its interaction with CD28 (present on T-cells). This interaction is a costimulatory signal necessary for adequate T-cell activation. Activated T cells have been shown to have an important role in the pathogenesis and the perpetuation of the inflammatory cascade in RA. Abatacept is therefore a selective costimulation modulator that inhibits T-cell activation. The most serious adverse reactions seen with abatacept are serious infections and malignancies. In particular, there are more cases of lung cancer observed with the use of this drug. In addition, the rate observed for lymphoma is approximately 3.5-fold higher than expected in an age- and gender-matched general population. Patients who have RA are considered to be at a higher risk for the development of lymphoma also, in particular patients who have active disease [34–37].

Rituximab is a chimeric monoclonal anti-CD20 antibody that depletes B cells. It has been approved for use in patients who have RA in combination with MTX. A study published in the *New England Journal of Medicine* in 2004 with Rituximab in patients who had RA showed a significant improvement after two infusions of Rituximab alone or in combination with MTX or cyclophosphamide [38]. It caused a decrease in B-cell numbers in peripheral blood for up to 24 weeks, without a significant decrease in total immunoglobulin levels. It also showed a decrease in rheumatoid factor levels.

Table 1 shows relevant aspects of the most commonly used antirheumatic drugs.

Use of cyclo-oxygenase-2–specific nonsteroidal anti-inflammatory drugs and cardiac risk

There has been in recent years a lot of controversy regarding the use of nonsteroidal anti-inflammatory drugs (NSAIDs), mainly with respect to safety issues and particularly cardiovascular risks with cyclo-oxygenase-2 (COX-2) inhibitors. Some studies have shown that COX-2 inhibitors, particularly celecoxib, do not have a significantly increased risk for cardiovascular events when compared with other nonselective NSAIDs and/or similar risk to placebo [39–44]. Based on these data, celecoxib, a selective COX-2 inhibitor, and nonselective NSAIDs carry a similar risk for cardiovascular events. On the other hand, other studies have shown a dose-related increased risk for cardiovascular events with COX-2 inhibitors. This risk was shown in two studies published in the *New England Journal of Medicine* last year, in which celecoxib was used for colorectal adenomas and adenomatous polyp prevention [45–46]. Based on this information, it is advisable to use these drugs for symptomatic relief in patients who have RA who are in the process of waiting for DMARDs to take effect. In general it is recommended to limit their use and to advise patients who have RA to use them only on an as-needed basis, because they do not have effects on prevention of disease progression. The choice between using a nonselective NSAID versus a COX-2 inhibitor should still be based on gastrointestinal side-effect risks for the individual patient. An important factor is to discuss with patients the risks involved and instruct them on the importance of avoiding chronic therapy with NSAIDs if unnecessary. Also it must be taken into consideration the patient's confidence in taking the medication to assure compliance when needed. If the choice is a nonselective NSAID and there is a need for prolonged therapy, it is recommended to combine it with a proton pump inhibitor, which has been shown to have some protective effects on gastrointestinal complications. The recommendation is to limit the use of these medications to the shortest possible period of time and at the lowest effective dose.

Perioperative management of antirheumatic drug therapy

Antirheumatic drugs can suppress inflammatory and immune responses needed for adequate wound healing and to fight infections [47,48]. Another important aspect in the management of patients who have rheumatoid arthritis therefore is the perioperative use of antirheumatic drugs to minimize perioperative and postoperative complications. To date there are not enough evidence-based data to establish a specific algorithm to follow in this setting, but some general guidelines are available based on the current data and mechanisms of action of these drugs.

Studies undertaken using MTX during the perioperative period have been confounding. For example, in a small retrospective study published in the *Journal of Rheumatology*, 38 patients were divided into those who had discontinued MTX therapy less than 4 weeks before surgery and those who had discontinued it 4 weeks or more before their elective procedure [49]. In this study there were four patients who had complications in the first group versus none in the second group. Complications included infections and wound dehiscence. Several studies, however, including two prospective trials, have shown no significant adverse effects in the recovery period after orthopedic surgery when MTX is continued perioperatively [50–56]. In fact, some have shown a decreased incidence in flares of the arthritis. The larger

Table 1
Anti-rheumatic drugs pearls

Medication	Usual dosing	Pre-monitoring	Regular monitoring	Adverse reactions	Contraindication/warnings (partial/absolute)
Hydroxychloroquine (Plaquenil)	200 mg BID	Ophthalmology evaluation	Ophthalmology evaluation every 6 months to 1 year	GI upset, visual loss	Retinal or visual field changes attributable to any 4-aminoquinoline compound, known hypersensitivity
SSA	1–3 g divided BID	CBC with WBC count differential and LFTs	CBC with WBC count differential and LFTs regularly; creatinine, UA	GI upset, rash, BM suppression, elevated liver enzymes, renal damage	Allergy to sulfa
MTX	7.5–20 mg PO weekly or up to 25 mg parenterally	Hepatitis screen, CBC with WBC count differential and LFTs, creatinine	CBC with WBC count differential and LFTs regularly; creatinine, UA	GI upset, malaise, fatigue, fever, ulcerative stomatitis, leucopenia, aplastic anemia, pancytopenia, hepatotoxicity, infection, interstitial pneumonitis, renal failure, skin rash	Pregnant women, nursing mothers, patients who have alcoholism or alcoholic or chronic liver disease, immunodeficiency syndromes, pre-existing blood dyscrasias, or hypersensitivity to MTX

TNF-inhibitors Etanercept (Enbrel) Adalimumab (Humira) Remicade (Infliximab)	50 mg SC once a week; 40 mg SC every 2 weeks; 3 mg/kg at 0, 2, and 6 weeks and then every 8 weeks	PPD (tuberculin) skin test	None	Infections, demyelinating disease/MS, lupus-like syndrome, cytopenias, ± neoplasia/ lymphoma, worsening CHF, injection site reactions/infusion reactions	MS, ± SLE, CHF
Abatacept (Orencia)	<60 kg, 500 mg 60–100 kg, 750 mg >100 kg, 1g	PPD (tuberculin) skin test	None	Common: headaches, URTI, nausea Serious: severe infection and malignancies	Known hypersensitivity to Orencia, concomitant use of TNF-inhibitors

Abbreviations: BID, twice daily; BM, bone marrow; CBC, complete blood count; CHF, congestive heart failure; GI, gastrointestinal; LFTs, liver function tests; MS, multiple sclerosis; PO, orally; SC, subcutaneously; SLE, systemic lupus erythematosus; UA, urinalysis; URTI, upper respiratory tract infections; WBC, white blood cells.

of the prospective trials had 388 patients who had RA and who were undergoing elective orthopedic surgery; it showed no significant increase in infection or delayed wound healing.

A study published in *Foot and Ankle International* in 2000 looked at the infectious and healing complications after elective orthopedic foot and ankle surgery using TNF-inhibitor therapy and concluded that TNF-inhibitors could be safely administered in the perioperative period without increasing the risk for infections or healing complications [57]. This was also the case in another small retrospective study in which those who continued therapy with TNF-inhibitors did not show an increase in complications as compared with those who stopped therapy perioperatively [58]. In contrast to these results, a more recent study published last year in *Arthritis and Rheumatism* showed a significant increase in serious infections in patients using TNF-inhibitor therapy [59].

There is limited data on the perioperative use of other antirheumatic agents, including leflunomide, SSA, azathioprine, and hydroxychloroquine. There was a retrospective study that looked at the effects of different DMARDs, including gold salts, MTX, azathioprine, SSA, hydroxychloroquine, and D-penicillamine on early wound complications and found no statistically significant increased risk for postoperative complications with gold salts, hydroxychloroquine, or SSA [51]. A more recent study investigating Leflunomide showed an increased incidence of postoperative wound healing complications compared with MTX and recommended that it should be stopped perioperatively [60]. Hydroxychloroquine is considered safe to be continued perioperatively. Leflunomide, SSA, and azathioprine should be held before surgery because of their possible toxicities.

References

[1] Harris ED Jr, Budd RC, Firestein GS, et al. Kelley's textbook of rheumatology. 7th edition. Elsevier Saunders; 2005. p. 996.
[2] Raza K, Breese M, Nightingale P, et al. Predictive value of antibodies to cyclic citrullinated peptide in patients with very early inflammatory arthritis. J Rheumatol 2005;32:231–8.
[3] Lee DM, Schur PH. Clinical utility of the anti-CCP assay in patients with rheumatic diseases. Ann Rheum Dis 2003;62:870.
[4] Zeng X, Ai M, Tian X, et al. Diagnostic value of anti-cyclic citrullinated peptide antibody in patients with rheumatoid arthritis. J Rheumatol 2003;30:1451.
[5] Van Gaalen FA, Linn-Rasker SP, van Venrooij WJ, et al. Autoantibodies to cyclic citrullinated peptides predicts progression to rheumatoid arthritis in patients with undifferentiated arthritis. Arthritis Rheum 2004;50:709.
[6] Arnett FC, Edworthy SM, Bloch DA, et al. The American Rheumatism Association 1987 Revised Criteria for the Classification of Rheumatoid Arthritis. Arthritis Rheum 1988;31:315–24.
[7] Prescribing information, Sulfasalazine delayed release tablets, USP (Azulfidine EN-tabs ®). Pharmacia & Upjohn Company, Division of Pfizer Inc. New York, New York; 2006.
[8] Kremer JM, Alarcón GS, Lightfoot RW, et al. Methotrexate for rheumatoid arthritis: Suggested guidelines for monitoring liver toxicity. Arthritis Rheum 1994;3:316.
[9] Prescribing information, Methotrexate sodium tablets (Rheumatrex ®). Heumann Pharma Gmblt, for Stada Pharmaceuticals Inc, Cranbury, New Jersey; 2003.

[10] O'Dell JR, Leff R, Paulsen G, et al. Treatment of rheumatoid arthritis with methotrexate and hydroxychloroquine, methotrexate and sulfasalazine, or a combination of the three medications: results of a two-year, randomized, double-blind, placebo-controlled trial. Arthritis Rheum 2002;46:1164.

[11] O'Dell JR, Haire CE, Erikson N, et al. Treatment of rheumatoid arthritis with methotrexate alone, sulfasalazine and hydroxychloroquine, or a combination of all three medications. N Engl J Med 1996;334:1287.

[12] Montesinos MC, Desai A, Delano D, et al. Adenosine A2A or A3 receptors are required for inhibition of inflammation by methotrexate and its analog MX-68. Arthritis Rheum 2003; 48:240.

[13] Cronstein BN, Naime D, Ostad E. The anti-inflammatory mechanism of methotrexate: increased adenosine release at inflamed sites diminishes leukocyte accumulation in an in vivo model of inflammation. J Clin Invest 1993;2675–82.

[14] Prescribing information. Etanercept (Enbrel®) Immunex Corporation, Thousand Oaks, California; 2006.

[15] Prescribing information. Infliximab (Remicade®) Centocor Inc.; 2006.

[16] Prescribing information. Adalimumab (Humira®) Abbott Laboratories, North Chicago, Illinois; 2006.

[17] Moreland LW, Baumgatner SW, Schiff MH, et al. Treatment of rheumatoid arthritis with a recombinant tumor necrosis factor receptor (p75)-Fc fusion protein. N Engl J Med 1997;337:141.

[18] Moreland LW, Schiff MH, Baumgartner SW, et al. Etanercept therapy in rheumatoid arthritis. A randomized, controlled trial. Ann Intern Med 1999;130:478.

[19] Weinblatt MH, Kremer JM, Bankhurst AD, et al. A trial of etanercept, a TNF receptor: Fc fusion protein in patients with rheumatoid arthritis receiving methotrexate. N Engl J Med 1999;340:253.

[20] Moreland LW, Cohen SB, Baumgartner SW, et al. Long-term safety and efficacy of etanercept in patients with rheumatoid arthritis. J Rheumatol 2001;28:1238.

[21] Bathon JM, Martin RW, Fleischmann RM, et al. A comparison of etanercept and methotrexate in patients with early rheumatoid arthritis. N Engl J Med 2000;343:1586.

[22] Petersen K, Leff R, Paulsen G, et al. Etanercept in combination with sulfasalazine (SSA), hydroxychloroquine (HCQ), or gold in the treatment of rheumatoid arthritis (RA) [abstract]. Arthritis Rheum 2003;48:S324.

[23] Maini R, St. Clair EW, Breedveld F, et al. Infliximab (chimeric anti-tumour necrosis factor alpha monoclonal antibody) versus placebo in rheumatoid arthritis patients receiving concomitant methotrexate: a randomized phase III trial. Lancet 1999;354:1932.

[24] Lipsky PE, van der Heijde DM, St Clair EW, et al. Infliximab and methotrexate in the treatment of rheumatoid arthritis. Anti-Tumor Necrosis Factor Trial in Rheumatoid Arthritis with Concomitant Therapy Study Group. N Engl J Med 2000;343:1594.

[25] Maini RN, Breedveld FC, Kalden JR, et al. Sustained improvement over two years in physical function, structural damage, and signs and symptoms among patients with rheumatoid arthritis treated with infliximab and methotrexate. Arthritis Rheum 2004;50:1051.

[26] Breedveld FC, Emery P, Keystone E, et al. Infliximab in active early rheumatoid arthritis. Ann Rheum Dis 2004;63:149.

[27] St Clair EW, Wagner CL, Fasanmade AA, et al. The relationship of serum infliximab concentrations to clinical improvement in rheumatoid arthritis: results from ATTRACT, a multicenter, randomized, double-blind, placebo-controlled trial. Arthritis Rheum 2002;46:1451.

[28] Westhovens R, Yocum D, Han J, et al. The safety of infliximab, combined with background treatments, among patients with rheumatoid arthritis and various comorbidities: a large, randomized, placebo-controlled trial. Arthritis Rheum 2006;54:1075.

[29] St Clair EW, van der Heijde DM, Smolen JS, et al. Combination of infliximab and methotrexate therapy for early rheumatoid arthritis: a randomized, controlled trial. Arthritis Rheum 2004;50:3432.

[30] Weinblatt ME, Keystone EC, Furst DE, et al. Adalimumab, a fully human anti-tumor necrosis factor alpha monoclonal antibody, for the treatment of rheumatoid arthritis in patients taking concomitant methotrexate: the ARMADA trial. Arthritis Rheum 2003;48:35.

[31] van de Putte LB, Atkins C, Malaise M, et al. Efficacy and safety of adalimumab as monotherapy in patients with rheumatoid arthritis for whom previous disease modifying antirheumatic drug treatment has failed. Ann Rheum Dis 2004;63:508.

[32] Keystone EC, Kavanaugh AF, Sharp JT, et al. Radiographic, clinical, and functional outcomes of treatment with adalimumab (a human anti-tumor necrosis factor monoclonal antibody) in patients with active rheumatoid arthritis receiving concomitant methotrexate therapy: a randomized, placebo-controlled, 52-week trial. Arthritis Rheum 2004;50:1400.

[33] Breedveld FC, Weisman MH, Kavanaugh AF, et al. The PREMIER study: a multicenter, randomized, double-blind clinical trial of combination therapy with adalimumab plus methotrexate versus methotrexate alone or adalimumab alone in patients with early, aggressive rheumatoid arthritis who had not had previous methotrexate treatment. Arthritis Rheum 2006;54:26.

[34] Prescribing information. Abatacept (Orencia®) Bristol-Myers Squibb Company, Princeton, New Jersey; 2007.

[35] Kremer JM, Westhovens R, Leon MMD, et al. Treatment of rheumatoid arthritis by selective inhibition of T-cell activation with fusion protein CTLA4Ig. N Engl J Med 2003;349:1907–15.

[36] Kremer JM, Dougados M, Emery P, et al. Treatment of rheumatoid arthritis with the selective costimulation modulator abatacept: twelve-month results of a phase IIb, double-blind, randomized, placebo-controlled trial. Arthritis Rheum 2005;52:2263.

[37] Westhovens R, Cole JC, Li T, et al. Improved health-related quality of life for rheumatoid arthritis patients treated with abatacept who have inadequate response to anti-TNF therapy in a double-blind, placebo-controlled, multicentre randomized clinical trial. Rheumatology (Oxford) 2006;45:1238–46.

[38] Edwards JC, Szczepanski L, Szechinski J, et al. Efficacy of B-cell-targeted therapy with rituximab in patients with rheumatoid arthritis. N Engl J Med 2004;350:2572.

[39] Graham DJ, Campen D, Hui R, et al. Risk of acute myocardial infarction and sudden cardiac death in patients treated with cyclo-oxygenase 2 selective and non-selective non-steroidal anti-inflammatory drugs: nested case-control study. Lancet 2005;365:475.

[40] Levesque LE, Brophy JM, Zhang B. Time variations in the risk of myocardial infarction among elderly users of COX-2 inhibitors. CMAJ 2006;174:1563.

[41] Silverstein FE, Faich G, Goldstein JL, et al. Gastrointestinal toxicity with celecoxib vs nonsteroidal anti-inflammatory drugs for osteoarthritis and rheumatoid arthritis. The CLASS study: a randomized controlled trial. JAMA 2000;284:1247.

[42] White WB, Faich G, Borer JS, et al. Cardiovascular thrombotic events in arthritis trials of the cyclooxygenase-2 inhibitor celecoxib. Am J Cardiol 2003;92:411.

[43] Singh G, Fort JG, Goldstein JL, et al. Celecoxib versus naproxen and diclofenac in osteoarthritis patients: SUCCESS-I Study. Am J Med 2006;119:255.

[44] Andersohn F, Schade R, Suissa S, et al. Cyclooxygenase-2 selective nonsteroidal antiinflammatory drugs and the risk of ischemic stroke: a nested case-control study. Stroke 2006;37:1725.

[45] Bertagnolli MM, Eagle CJ, Zauber AG, et al. Celecoxib for the prevention of sporadic colorectal adenomas. N Engl J Med 2006;355:873.

[46] Arber N, Eagle CJ, Spicak J, et al. Celecoxib for the prevention of colorectal adenomatous polyps. N Engl J Med 2006;355:885.

[47] Busti AJ, Hooper JS, Amaya CJ, et al. Effects of perioperative antiinflammatory and immunomodulating therapy on surgical wound healing. Pharmacotherapy 2005;25(11):1566–91.

[48] Jain A, Maini R, Nanchahal J. Disease modifying treatment and elective surgery in rheumatoid arthritis: the need for more data. Ann Rheum Dis 2004;63:602.

[49] Bridges SL Jr, Lopez-Mendez A, Han KH, et al. Should methotrexate be discontinued before elective orthopedic surgery in patients with rheumatoid arthritis? J Rheumatol 1991; 18:984.

[50] Carpenter MT, West SG, Vogelgesang SA, et al. Postoperative joint infections in rheumatoid arthritis patients on methotrexate therapy. Orthopedics 1996;19:207.

[51] Escalante A, Beardmore TD. Risk factors for early wound complications after orthopedic surgery for rheumatoid arthritis. J Rheumatol 1995;22:1844.

[52] Grennan DM, Gray J, Loudon J, et al. Methotrexate and early postoperative complications in patients with rheumatoid arthritis undergoing elective orthopaedic surgery. Ann Rheum Dis 2001;60:214–7.

[53] Jain A, Witbreuk M, Ball C, et al. Influence of steroids and methotrexate on wound complications after elective rheumatoid hand and wrist surgery. J Hand Surg [Am] 2002;27:449–55.

[54] Kasdan ML, June L. Postoperative results of rheumatoid arthritis patients on methotrexate at the time of reconstructive surgery of the hand. Orthopedics 1993;16:1233.

[55] Perhala RS, Wilke WS, Clough JD, et al. Local infectious complications following large joint replacement in rheumatoid arthritis patients treated with methotrexate versus those not treated with methotrexate. Arthritis Rheum 1991;34:146.

[56] Sany J, Anaya JM, Canovas F, et al. Influence of methotrexate on the frequency of postoperative infectious complications in patients with rheumatoid arthritis. J Rheumatol 1993;20: 1129–32.

[57] Bibbo C, Goldberg JW. Infectious and healing complications after elective orthopaedic foot and ankle surgery during tumor necrosis factor-alpha inhibition therapy. Foot Ankle Int 2004;25:331–5.

[58] Talwalkar SC, Grennan DM, Gray J, et al. Tumour necrosis factor alpha antagonists and early postoperative complications in patients with inflammatory joint disease undergoing elective orthopaedic surgery. Ann Rheum Dis 2005;64:650.

[59] Giles JT, Bartlett SJ, Gelber AC, et al. Tumor necrosis factor inhibitor therapy and risk of serious postoperative orthopedic infection in rheumatoid arthritis. Arthritis Rheum 2006;55: 333.

[60] Fuerst M, Mohl H, Baumgartel K, et al. Leflunomide increased the risk of early healing complications in patients with rheumatoid arthritis undergoing elective orthopedic surgery. Rheumatol Int 2006;26(12):1138–42.

FOOT AND ANKLE CLINICS

Index

Note: Page numbers of article titles are in **boldface** type.

metatarsophalangeal joint and,
impairment of, 442–444
improvement of, 449
nonpreservation surgery versus,
440, 450–451
on first rays, 437, 439–440
arthrodesis role in, 451–452
results of, 441–443, 448–449
on lateral rays, 440–441
results of, 443–445, 449
on lesser rays, 438–440, 446–447
resection arthroplasty role
in, 451–452
results of, 445
postoperative protocol for,
441–442
preoperative status of, 436,
439–440
specific problems encountered
with, 450–451
study methods for, 436–437
summary overview of, 435–436,
452–453
technique principles for, 437–440

K

Kates procedure, for metatarsal head
resection, 420–421

Keller procedure, for metatarsal head
resection, great toe, 407–408
lesser toes, 421

Kirschner wires, for rheumatoid forefoot
surgery, in hallux metatarsophalangeal
arthrodesis, 399–401
in metatarsal head resection,
420–421, 423, 426–428,
430–431
joint-preserving, 439, 441–442

L

Larmon procedure, for metatarsal head
resection, 421–422

Lateral rays, joint-preserving surgery on,
for rheumatoid forefoot, 440–441
results of, 443–445, 449

Leflunomide (Arava), for rheumatoid
arthritis, 527, 529
in ankle, 477–478
wound healing complications
associated with, 512, 514

Lesser rays/toes, joint-preserving surgery
on, for rheumatoid forefoot, 438–440,
446–447
resection arthroplasty role
in, 451–452

results of, 445
rheumatoid arthritis surgery of,
417–433
anatomic deformity and, 418–420
authors' preferred technique for,
423–430
complications of, 431
historical aspects of, 420–421
overview of, 417–418, 432
pathologic basis of, 418–420
results of, 430–431
theoretic basis of, 421–423

Lipscomb procedure, for metatarsal head
resection, 421–422

M

Magnetic resonance imaging (MRI), in
rheumatoid arthritis, for hindfoot
assessment, 457, 462
for total ankle replacement, 499

Malleolar fracture, in total ankle
replacement, 502, 505

Malunion, in ankle arthrodesis, for
rheumatoid arthritis, 491–492

Mayo resection, in hallux
metatarsophalangeal arthrodesis, for
rheumatoid forefoot, 398

Medical management, of rheumatoid
arthritis, in ankle, arthrodesis versus,
477–478
in hallux metatarsophalangeal
joint, 398, 406

Metatarsal curve, in joint-preserving
surgery, for rheumatoid forefoot,
449–450

Metatarsal formula, in joint-preserving
surgery, for rheumatoid forefoot,
437–439

Metatarsal head, in joint-preserving
surgery, for rheumatoid forefoot,
impairment of, 442–445
reconstruction of, 449
resection of, **417–433**
anatomic deformity
and, 418–420
authors' preferred technique for,
423–430
complications of, 431
historical aspects of, 420–421
overview of, 417–418, 432
pathologic basis of, 418–420
results of, 430–431
theoretic basis of, 421–423

P

Pain, rheumatoid arthritis causing, assessment of, 527
  management of, 527, 532–533

Pain control, for rheumatoid arthritis surgery, 520

Pale toe, intra-operative management of, 516, 518

Pannus formation, in rheumatoid forefoot, 418

Physical function, assessment of, in rheumatoid arthritis, 526–527

Pin fixation, in arthrodesis, for rheumatoid hindfoot, 468
  of hallux metatarsophalangeal joint, of rheumatoid forefoot, 399–400
  in metatarsal head resection, 428
  retrograde, digital perfusion and, 519–520
  removal of, 522

Plantar approach, to metatarsal head resection, 420–421, 425

Plantar fasciitis, in rheumatoid hindfoot, 457, 459–460

Plantar fat pad, in rheumatoid forefoot, 419–420

Posterior tibial tendon dysfunction (PTTD), in rheumatoid hindfoot, diagnosis of, 458, 461
  management of, 461–463

Preoperative evaluation, for rheumatoid arthritis surgery, 510–512
  of ankle, 498–500
  of forefoot, 436, 439–440

Prostheses, for total ankle replacement, 504
  STAR implant, 470, 502–506
  TNK implant, 468–470, 504

PT/INR, rheumatoid arthritis surgery complications and, 519, 521, 523

aPTT, rheumatoid arthritis surgery complications and, 519, 521, 523

Pulse volume recordings, in rheumatoid arthritis surgery, intraoperative measures of, 519–520
  preoperative evaluation of, 511

R

Radiographs, in rheumatoid arthritis, for hindfoot assessment, 457, 462

for total ankle replacement, 498–501

Reconstruction surgery, for rheumatoid forefoot, **405–416**. See also *Hallux metatarsophalangeal arthroplasty.*

Resection arthroplasty, of first metatarsal head, for rheumatoid arthritis, 406–410
  arthrodesis versus, 408–410
  Keller's procedure for, 407–408

Retrocalcaneal bursitis, in rheumatoid hindfoot, 457, 460

Revision arthroplasty, for rheumatoid forefoot, 429–430

Rheumatoid arthritis (RA), **525–537**
  characteristics of, 405–406, 525
  clinical course of, 476, 525
  diagnosis of, 526
  drug therapy for, algorithm for selection of, 527–529
    biologics as, 529–530
    cardiac risk with, 530–531
    cyclo-oxygenase-2-specific nonsteroidal anti-inflammatory drugs as, 530–531
    mechanism of action of, 529
    perioperative management of, 531, 534
    specific agents in, 527, 532–533
  of ankle, arthrodesis in, **475–495**
    arthroscopic technique for, 481
    author's preferred technique for, 483–490
    bimalleolar fracture and, 485–489
    clinical results of, 480–489
    complications of, 490–492
    compression screws for, 480–481, 485
    equipment set up for, 483–484, 488–489
    external fixation for, 481–482
    fibular strut graft for, 482, 484–487
    medical management considerations, 477–478
    osteoporosis and, 479–480
    overview of, 475–477, 492
    sliding bone graft for, 482
    soft-tissue disease and, 477, 479, 485–486, 488
  management of, **455–474,** 457

Moving?

Make sure your subscription moves with you!

To notify us of your new address, find your **Clinics Account Number** (located on your mailing label above your name), and contact customer service at:

E-mail: elspcs@elsevier.com

800-654-2452 (subscribers in the U.S. & Canada)
407-345-4000 (subscribers outside of the U.S. & Canada)

Fax number: 407-363-9661

Elsevier Periodicals Customer Service
6277 Sea Harbor Drive
Orlando, FL 32887-4800

*To ensure uninterrupted delivery of your subscription, please notify us at least 4 weeks in advance of move.